Fore

M

GW01417372

System requirement:
- **Windows XP or above**
- **Power DVD player (Software)**
- **Windows media player 10.0 version or above (Software)**

Accompanying Photo CD ROM is playable only in Computer and not in DVD player.

Kindly wait for few seconds for Photo CD to autorun. If it does not autorun then please do the following:
- Click on my computer
- Click the **drive labelled JAYPEE** and after opening the drive, kindly double click the file **Jaypee**

Forensic Radiology Made Easy®

D Govindiah

Professor and Head (Retd)
Department of Forensic Medicine
Osmania Medical College
Hyderabad, Andhra Pradesh, India

Foreword
C Ramachandran

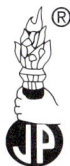

JAYPEE BROTHERS MEDICAL PUBLISHERS (P) LTD

Hyderabad • St Louis (USA) • Panama City (Panama) • London (UK) • New Delhi
Ahmedabad • Bengaluru • Chennai • Kochi • Kolkata • Lucknow • Mumbai • Nagpur

Published by

Jitendar P Vij

Jaypee Brothers Medical Publishers (P) Ltd

Corporate Office

4838/24 Ansari Road, Daryaganj, **New Delhi** - 110002, India
Phone: +91-11-43574357, Fax: +91-11-43574314

Registered Office

B-3 EMCA House, 23/23B Ansari Road, Daryaganj, **New Delhi** - 110 002, India
Phones: +91-11-23272143, +91-11-23272703, +91-11-23282021, +91-11-23245672
Rel: +91-11-32558559, Fax: +91-11-23276490, +91-11-23245683
e-mail: jaypee@jaypeebrothers.com, Website: www.jaypeebrothers.com

Offices in India

- **Ahmedabad**, Phone: Rel: +91-79-32988717, e-mail: ahmedabad@jaypeebrothers.com
- **Bengaluru**, Phone: Rel: +91-80-32714073, e-mail: bangalore@jaypeebrothers.com
- **Chennai**, Phone: Rel: +91-44-32972089, e-mail: chennai@jaypeebrothers.com
- **Hyderabad**, Phone: Rel:+91-40-32940929, e-mail: hyderabad@jaypeebrothers.com
- **Kochi**, Phone: +91-484-2395740, e-mail: kochi@jaypeebrothers.com
- **Kolkata**, Phone: +91-33-22276415, e-mail: kolkata@jaypeebrothers.com
- **Lucknow**, Phone: +91-522-3040554, e-mail: lucknow@jaypeebrothers.com
- **Mumbai**, Phone: Rel: +91-22-32926896, e-mail: mumbai@jaypeebrothers.com
- **Nagpur**, Phone: Rel: +91-712-3245220, e-mail: nagpur@jaypeebrothers.com

Overseas Offices

- **North America Office, USA,** Ph: 001-636-6279734
  e-mail: jaypee@jaypeebrothers.com, anjulav@jaypeebrothers.com
- **Central America Office, Panama City, Panama**
  Ph: 001-507-317-0160, e-mail: cservice@jphmedical.com
  Website: www.jphmedical.com
- **Europe Office, UK,** Ph: +44 (0) 2031708910
  e-mail: info@jpmedpub.com

Forensic Radiology Made Easy®

© 2011, Jaypee Brothers Medical Publishers

This book has been published in good faith that the material provided by author is original. Every effort is made to ensure accuracy of material, but the publisher, printer and author will not be held responsible for any inadvertent error(s). In case of any dispute, all legal matters are to be settled under Delhi jurisdiction only.

First Edition: 2003
Second Edition: **2011**

ISBN 978-93-5025-036-5

Typeset at JPBMP typesetting unit

Printed at Rajkamal Electric Press, Plot No. 2, Phase-IV, Kundli, Haryana.

To
my eldest brother Venkatesam
and
his wife Rangamma

Foreword

It gives me immense pleasure to write the foreword for *Forensic Radiology Made Easy*® based on rich experience of many years of the author in determining the age from X-rays and other aspects of forensic radiology. The introduction to anatomical aspects in the preliminary pages in a very simple style has been written considering the need of this essential basic knowledge in dealing with the medicolegal work especially when it involves X-rays. I am of the firm opinion that *Forensic Radiology Made Easy*® will be helpful to medical men; law enforcing officers, and law courts in solving complex legal problems. It is the work of appreciation produced by Dr D Govindiah in a simple way to help the doctors facing complex medico-legal problems. The author is a popular professor of forensic medicine and medicolegal expert, who helped in many puzzled medicolegal problems in various states. It is a dedicated work based on long experience and indeed a commendable job done to educate the medical doctors and the medical students. I am sure it will prove success in its fulfilment.

C Ramachandran
Dean
Vinayaka Mission's Medical College and Hospital
Karaikal, Union Territory of Pondicherry, India

Preface to
the Second Edition

It gives me immense pleasure in bringing out the second edition of my earlier book *Forensic Radiology Made Easy*® through one of the leading medical publishers, M/s Jaypee Brothers Medical Publishers, who has of late carved a special name for themselves in the field of medical publishing.

The first edition which was published long ago which is very concise in nature and served its purpose of emphasizing the value of skiagrams in the study and of appearance of ossification centers and their fusion especially with the shafts of long bones around the various large joints in the living which would help in determining the age of the individuals.

Keeping the need of the hour in mind, this thoroughly revised edition is being brought out which would come in handy in dealing with especially the medicolegal cases, its thorough examinations and further certification to solve the numerous legal problems in the courts of law.

With the addition of entirely new chapters viz, Exercises for Age Estimation, Radiographic Positioning, and Radiology and Firearm Injuries and the ample of new illustrations and drawings, this second edition would be of immense value to the practicing doctors, law enforcing authorities, medical students both undergraduates and postgraduates who are pursuing in special interest in the fields of Forensic Medicine and Toxicology and Radiology.

D Govindiah

Preface to the First Edition

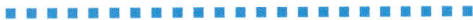

In writing this concise edition of *Forensic Radiology* which includes *Radiological Age Determination* and fractures of bones of medicolegal importance, my basic aim is to emphasize the value of skiagrams in the study and of appearance of ossification centers and their fusion, especially with the shafts of long bones around the various large joints in the living which would help in determining the age of the individual. This need is much more felt in dealing with the medicolegal cases in their examinations and certification to solve the various legal problems in the courts of law. Now the radiological examinations are the recognized scientific methods for the courts and in solving complex problems of litigation. In this volume each radiograph is accompanied by a line drawing of the same to explain the reader of the proper subject and highlight the salient features present on the X-ray film. Forensic medicine is a complex specialty facing complex problems to be solved in a legal way. The plain X-ray material used in compiling the concise book is from Osmania Medical College, Gandhi Medical College and Vinayaka Mission's Medical College, Departments of Forensic Medicine and VM Hospital. Anteroposterior (AP) and posteroanterior (PA) and lateral views of major joints and of other parts have been used in the study. The ossification centers of both proximal and distal ends of long bones in the living; their appearance and fusion at different stages with their shafts and different periods of ages have been studied. The traumatic bone injuries in medicolegal cases and other cases of medicolegal importance have been added to make the volume more interesting.

Though more advance modern techniques like ultrasound, CT and MRI are available, but they are of no added value when compared to the plain X-rays. The purpose of this volume is to educate the doctors, law enforcing authorities and also to form source reference to them in complex issues to solve medicolegal problems. Many years of experience in medicolegal work has been reflected by the author in the volume to interpret and solve the tricky problems in a more scientific way and depose their evidence on law requirements.

D Govindiah

Acknowledgments

My sincere gratitude to Dr C Ramachandran, MD, PhD, Dean, Vinayaka Mission's Medical College, Karaikal, Pondicherry for giving me constant encouragement in preparing the concise book.

I am grateful to Dr R Gandhi, MD, Principal, Vinayaka Mission's Medical College, Karaikal, Dr GR Bhaskar, Postgraduate Professor and HOD, Shadan Medical Institute, Hyderabad, Andhra Pradesh, Dr Susheela Rajendran Medical Superintendent, VMMC Hospital and Dr K Ramalingam, Chief Radiologist, Vinayaka Mission's Medical College, Karaikal, Pondicherry for the valuable guidance in bringing out *Forensic Radiology Made Easy*® of practical importance particularly to those of the medical profession.

The author is deeply indebted to the following esteemed colleagues who have helped in bringing out the book:
- Dr M Narayan Reddy
- Dr Surender Reddy
- Dr Chandre Gowda
- Dr Hari Krishna
- Dr M Shankar
- Dr R Ramchandra Rao

I am very thankful to receive extensive help from Mr P Muralidhar, Mr TR Saravanan, Miss J Suganthy, and Mrs Sandy who has compiled this work in computer.

I am thankful to the following esteemed colleagues for their valuable contribution and encouragement:
- Shri SA Chellappa
- Dr KS Narayan Reddy
- Dr A Ramesh
- Dr Dillip Kumar Suryawanshi
- Shri A Karthikeyan
- Miss M Hemamalini
- Dr G Chandrasekaran
- Dr Chandra Gowda
- Dr Sree Ramulu
- Dr M Shekhar
- Dr R Ramchander Rao
- Dr T Madan Mohan
- Dr D Ranganath Swamy
- Dr D Sangeeta
- Dr Padmasree

I express my sincere thanks to the following for their help in preparing the typescript:
- G Selvakumaran
- M Haji Mohamed

My special thanks to Shri Jitendar P Vij (Chairman and Managing Director) and Mr Tarun Duneja (Director-Publishing) of Jaypee Brothers Medical Publisher (P) Ltd and also author co-ordinator Mr Suresh (Hyderabad Branch).

Contents

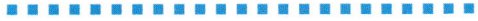

Introduction

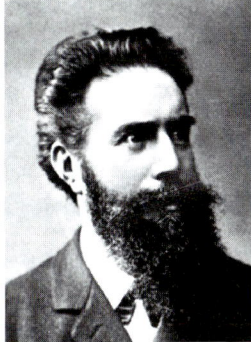

Wilhelm Roentgen (1845-1923)

Wilhelm Conrad Roentgen was born in a small German Village of Lennep. While he was studying in a local school, due to unknown reasons, he was expelled from the school and became a school dropout. But from the childhood his passion for science remained firm and did not fade away. As he was growing, he developed faith in the subjects of science and believed that the science was growing he developed all men and women and its application in everyday life could work wonders. His determination and aptitude for the science made him an assistant to the distinguished German Physicist August Kundt. After some efforts, he secured an appointment at the University of Warzburg and became the Head of Department in 1895, he accidentally discovered invisible X-rays, i.e. electromagnetic waves having short wavelength. When he exposed his hand to the beam of X-rays they passed through the flesh and where as the bones seen almost opaque and produced image of his own hand on fluorescent screen. He called his wife and asked her to place her left hand on the photographic plate and passed the beam of X-rays. A permanent image of the bones of her hand appeared along with her wedding ring on the plate. Thus, the first ever X-ray photograph in the world had been taken. Thus the era of imaging science had begun. Doctors could now look at what was inside the patient's inside and truthfully revealed many of the details. Apart from medical investigations, in other fields also the X-rays have made a remarkable contribution and the mankind together salutes Roentgen for this immense contribution to help reduce the sufferings of millions of patients world over. For this great contribution Roentgen

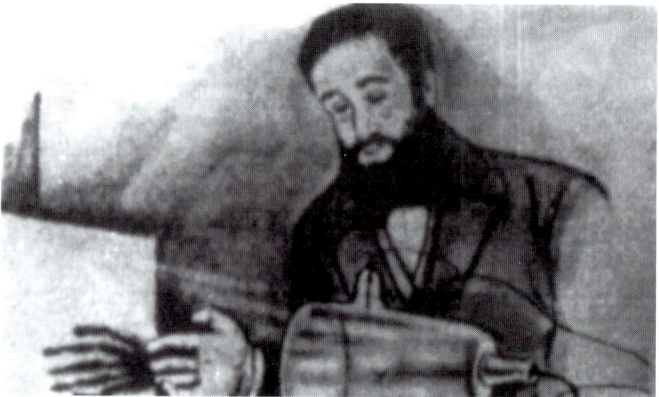

Prof Roentgen experimenting with the cathode ray tube, showing the bones of his hand on a photographic plate

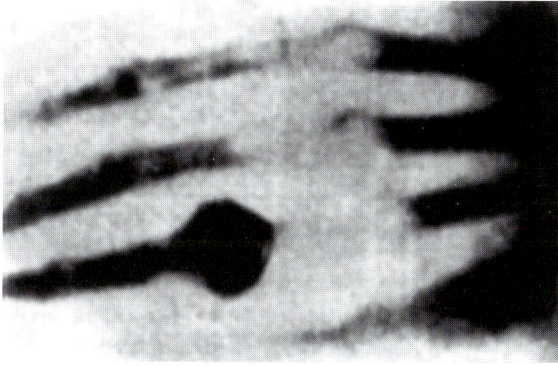

X-ray of Mrs Roentgen's hand.
Her diamond ring is visible as a shadow

was awarded the Noble prize in 1901. Now more than hundred years have passed since the discovery of X-rays and the discoverer has helped reduce the suffering since untold millions of mankind. Today other forms of imaging like ultrasound; magnetic resonance imaging (MRI) and CT scan are used but are expensive and not easily available.

Professor (Dr) Kakarla Subba Rao an authority on radiology is of view that the use of conventional radiological investigations should be used as far as possible as they are not costly; are easily available and more effective in diagnosis of fractures of bones and dislocations; infections of lungs; cancers of lung and kidney stones, etc.

THE MEDICAL IMAGING TECHNIQUES

They are simple radiography, CT scan; ultrasonography and MRI and other modern techniques.

SIMPLE RADIOGRAPHY

The simple radiography is the method in which the X-ray beam is passed through the patient on to a photographic plate; the short wavelengths of the X-rays penetrate and produce images of different densities. The dense tissue like the compact bone absorbs more X-rays than the less dense tissue of the spongy bone. The dense tissue produces transparent (white) areas on the X-ray film and the less dense tissue produces radiolucent (gray) areas. By using X-rays various view are taken by using methods of "Radiology of Positioning". In PA view, the X-rays traverse the patient from posterior to anterior side and in AP view the X-rays pass through the patient from anterior to posterior side. In lateral radiograph the lateral part of the body is placed close to the X-ray film while taking the X-ray.

Since the discovery of the X-rays in 1895, it has become possible to visualize the bones, joints, diseased internal organs and kidney and gallbladder's stones, etc. in the living individuals. Determining the age of a person by using plain X-rays in medico-legal cases and in other problems has become possible. The simple radiography has become the best method to visualize the appearance of ossification centers and their fusion to the shafts even though there are other modern imaging techniques like CT scan, ultrasonography and MRI available.

These modern methods are highly technical; require sophisticated machinery and are more complex and very expensive for a common man.

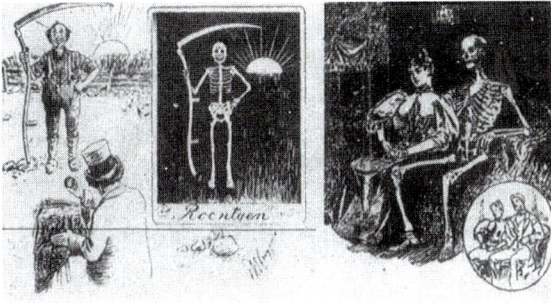

Roentgen photography—Smile Please!

COMPUTED TOMOGRAPHY (CT Scan)

This method, CT scan, shows radiographic images of the body that resemble transverse anatomical section. In this, the X-ray tube moves in an arc or circle around the body. The tube moves in one direction and the film on the opposite direction. Several films can be taken at the same time in a single exposure. These multitude of linear energy absorptions are measured and put into a computer. CT images are printouts from the computer. In this, e.g. the vertebrae are seen relatively transparent and those with little absorption as black.

ULTRASONOGRAPHY

Ultrasonography is the technique in which visualization of structures in the body by recording pulses of ultrasonic waves reflecting off the tissues. Echos from the body reflect into the transducer and convert to electrical energy. Electric signals are recorded and displayed on a TV monitor as a cross-sectional image recorded on videotape.

MAGNETIC RESONANCE IMAGING (MRI)

MRI shows images similar to that of CT scans.

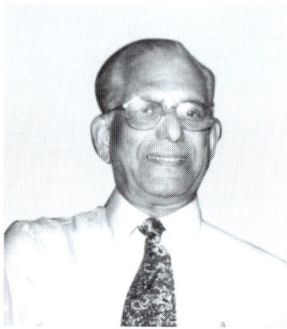

Prof Kakarla Subba Rao
Director, NIMS, Hyderabad

Prof Kakarla Subba Rao, an authority on radiology said that even today in any general hospital 80% of all investigations performed in radiology department are X-ray examinations. There are today other forms of imaging, which are used in the investigations like the ultrasound used in imaging the growth and development of the fetus. Ultrasonography has replaced X-ray in imaging to a large extent. However, X-rays made a come back in the computerized axial tomography (CAT). CT Scan has revolutionized the diagnostics of the brain and the spinal cord.

Another imaging technology that has been replacing the X-rays is the magnetic resonance imaging (MRI), but MRI is quite expensive and not so easily available.

Prof Kakarla Subba Rao feels that a tendency exists among the younger generation of doctors to investigate by using the latest high-tech gadgets. He feels however that they should resist this temptation and use the conventional radiological investigations as far as possible because the X-rays are a cost effective technology and are more effective in diagnosis of fractures, dislocations, infections of lung, kidney stones, cancers of lung and bones.

INDIAN PENAL CODE SECTIONS AND INDIAN ACTS

APPLICABLE IN AGES OF MEDICOLEGAL IMPORTANCE

1. *Sections of Indian Penal Code*

Section 82
Section 83 IPC
Section 87 IPC
Section 89 IPC
Section 361 IPC
Section 366-AIPC
Section 366-BIPC
Section 369
Section 375

2. *Indian Acts*

Indian Railway Act
Borastal School Act 1929
Juvenile Justice Act 1986
Indian Factory Act
Indian Majority Act 1875
Indian Evidence Act S.118
Childrens' Act 1960
Bombay Childrens' Act 1948
Child Marriage Restraint Act 1978
Indian Mines Act 1923
United Provinces Excise Act 1910
Indian Mines Act 1923, 1938

MEDICOLEGAL IMPORTANCE OF AGE AND THE LAW RELATING TO VARIOUS OFFENCES

Below 1 year	:	Section 300 IPC
		Section 302 IPC
		Infanticide
5 years	:	Criminal Act 1890
		Indian Railway Act, Responsibility for any Criminal Act
7 years	:	Section 82 IPC
		Criminal Act
7 years and under 12 years	:	Section 83 IPC
		Liability of juvenile offender.
10 years	:	Section 369 IPC
		Kidnapping (for movable property)
12 years	:	Responsibility for Criminal Acts. Consent for physical examination. Evidence in court of law. Valid consent to suffer any harm done in good faith.
14 years	:	Indian Factory Act – 1948
		For employment in a factory
15 years	:	Section 375 IPC
		Rape (Sexual intercourse)
16 years	:	Section 361 IPC
		Section 366-AIPC
		Section 366-BIPC
		Section 375 IPC
		Rape, kidnapping: A minor from lawful guardianship.
Consent	:	Juvenile and reformatory school

18 years	:	Indian Majority Act 1875 Attainment of majority civil and criminal responsibility. Kidnapping or abduction: A minor from lawful guardianship. Marriage contract (for female). Valid consent for surgical procedures. Right to cast vote. Above 18 years (female) mentally sound can make a valid will
21 years	:	Marriage contract (for male). Guardianship of court of wards. Stays of juvenile offender in a Borastal School who attains his age of majority at 21 years.
25-28 years	:	For entering into the Government service. Minimum age 18 years.
55-58 years	:	Age of retirement from Government services.
Above 65 years and above	:	Senior citizens for various concessions, e.g. railway traveling concessions and benefits.

SECTION 300 IPC

Murder

The act by which the death caused is done with intention of causing death, or

Secondly : If it is done with the intention of causing such bodily injury as the offender knows to be likely to cause the death of the person to whom the harm is caused, or

Thirdly: If it is done with the intention of causing bodily injury intended to be inflicted is sufficient in the ordinary course of nature to cause death, or

Fourthly : If the person committing the Act knows that it is so imminently dangerous that it must, in all probability, cause death, or such bodily injury as it likely to causing death or such injury as aforesaid.

SECTION 302 IPC

Punishment for Murder

Whoever commits murder shall be punished with death, or imprisonment for life, and shall also be liable to fine (infanticide is treated as murder in India).

SECTION 82 IPC

Act of child under seven years of age

Nothing is an offence, which is done by a child under 7 years of age (He cannot be convicted of crime).

Comment

A child below the age of 7 years cannot distinguish right from wrong.

A child under 7 years of age is liable to punishment under Railway Act (1890) if he does anything with malicious intent to wreck or attempt to wreck a train, to hurt or attempt to hurt persons traveling by railway or to endanger the safety of persons traveling by railway by willful act or by way of rash or negligent act or omission.

SECTION 83 IPC

Act of a child above 7 years and under 12 years of immature under standing. Nothing is an offence which is done by a child above 7 years of age and under 12 years, who has not attained sufficient maturity of understanding to judge the nature and consequences of his conduct on that occasion.

Comment

Where a child-accused over 7 years and below 12 years discloses an acute and intelligent mind, he must be held to know them.

SECTION 87 IPC

Act not intended and not known to be likely to cause death or grievous hurt, done by consent

Nothing which is not intended to cause death or grievous hurt and which is not known by the doer to be likely to cause death or grievous hurt, is an offence by reason of any harm which it may cause, or be intended by the doer to cause, to any person, above eighteen years of age, who has given consent, whether express or implied, to suffer that harm, or by reason of any harm which it may be known by the doer to be likely to cause to any such person who has consented to take the risk of that harm.

SECTION 89 IPC

Act done in good faith for benefit of child or insane person by or by consent of guardian

Nothing which is done in good faith for the benefit of a person under 12 years of age, or of unsound mind, or by consent either expressed or implied of the guardian or other person having lawful charge of that person, is an offence by reason of any harm, which it may cause or to be known by the doer to be likely to cause to that person provided.

PROVISOS

First

That this exception shall not extend to the intentional causing of death or to the attempting to cause death.

Second

That this exception shall not extend to the doing of anything, which the person doing it knows to be likely to cause death for any purpose other than the preventing of death or grievous hurt, or the curing of any grievous disease or infirmity.

Third

That this exception shall not extend to the voluntary causing of grievous hurt, or to the attempting to cause grievous hurt, unless it be for the purpose of preventing death or grievous hurt, or the curing of any grievous disease or infirmity.

Fourth

That this exception shall not extend to the abetment of any offence, to the committing of which it would not extend.

Comment

The section 89 IPC empowers the guarding of an infant under 12 years or of an insane person to consent, either expressly or impliedly to inflict harm on the infant, or the person, provided it is done in good faith and is done for his benefit.

(A child under 12 years of age cannot give valid consent to suffer any harm, which may occur from an act done in good faith)

SECTION 361 IPC

Kidnapping from lawful guardianship

Whoever takes or entices any minor under 16 years of age if a male or under 18 years if a female, or any person of unsound mind, out of the keeping of the lawful guardian of such minor or person of unsound mind without the consent of such guardian, is said to kidnap such minor or person from lawful guardianship

(The prosecution to prove that the girl is under the age of 21 years).

SECTION 366-A

Procuration of minor girl

Whoever, by any means whatsoever, induces any minor girl under the age of eighteen years to go from any place or to do any act with intent that such girl may be, or knowing that it is likely that she will be, forced or seduced to illicit intercourse with another person shall be punishable with imprisonment which may extend to 10 years, and shall also be liable to fine.

Comment

Ingredients to the offence under section: 366-A
1. That a minor girl below the age of 18 years is induced by the accused.

2. That she is induced to go from any place or to do any act, and
3. That she so induced with intent that she may be or knowing that it is likely that she will be forced or seduced to illegal intercourse with another person.

SECTION 366-B

Importation of girl from foreign country

Whoever imports into India from any country outside India or from the state of Jammu and Kashmir any girl under the age of 21 years with intent that she may be, or knowing it to be likely that she will be, forced or seduced to illicit intercourse with any person shall be punishable with imprisonment which may extend to ten years and shall also be liable to fine.

SECTION 369 IPC

Kidnapping or abducting child under 10 years with intent to steal from its person

Whoever kidnaps or abducts any child under the age of 10 years with the intention of taking dishonestly any movable property from the person of such child shall be punished with imprisonment of either description for a term which may extend to 7 years and shall also be liable to fine.

SECTION 375 IPC

Rape (Sexual Offence)

A man is said to commit "Rape" who except in the case here in after excepted, has sexual intercourse with a woman under circumstances falling under any of the six following descriptions.

First

Against her will

Second

Without her consent

Third

With her consent, when her consent has been obtained by putting her or any person in whom she is interested in fear of death, or of hurt.

Fourth

With her consent, when the man knows that he is not her husband, and that her consent is given because she believed that he is another man to whom she is or believes herself to be lawfully married.

Fifth

With her consent, when, at the time of giving such consent by reason of unsoundness of mind or intoxication or the administration by him personally or through another of any stupefying or unwholesome substance, she is unable to understand the nature and consequences of that to which she gives consent.

Sixth

With or without her consent when she is under sixteen years of age.

SECTION 375 IPC

Sexual intercourse by a man with a girl under 15 years of age, even if she be his own wife constitutes rape.

Any other girl under 16 years of age even with her consent, constitutes rape.

To constitute an offence of kidnapping or abducting, a minor from lawful guardianship, the age of a body should be under sixteen years and that of a girl under eighteen years.

INDIAN FACTORY ACT 1948

A child below the age of 14 years shall not be employed to work in any factory or mine or engaged in other hazardous employment.

No child who has not completed his 14th year shall be required or allowed to work in a factory.

A child who has completed his 14 years or an adolescent, shall not be required or allowed to work in a factory unless a certificate of fitness granted to him by a certifying surgeon is in the custody of the manager of the factory and such a child or adolescent carries, while he is at work, a token giving a reference to such a certificate (as per the Indian constitution a child below the age of 14 years shall not be employed to work in any factory or mine or engaged in hazardous employment).

Under the factory act 1948, a "Child" is defined as a person who has not completed his 15 years. No child shall be employed or permitted to work in a factory for more than four-and-a half hours in a day and between the hours of 7 pm and 6 am.

BORASTAL SCHOOL ACT 1929

The State Government may order a youthful offender who has attained the age of 16 years detained in a certified school to be transferred to a Borastal school established under the Borastal School Act 1929 in the interest of discipline or for other reasons.

'Youthful offender' means any child who has been found to have committed an offence and who shall not be sentenced to death or life imprisonment or imprisonment. A child charged with the commission of an offence shall be tried by a court of chief judicial magistrate or in any court specially empowered under the Childrens' Act 1960 or any other law for the time being inforce providing for the treatment, training and rehabilitation of youthful offenders and no conviction may be sent to a certified school but must not be detained there beyond the age of 18 years. A youthful offender is over the age of 14 years, the offender may be ordered to pay the fine.

INDIAN MAJORITY ACT 1875

A person is deemed to have attained his majority on the completion of 18 years which is assumes full civil rights and responsibilities (where a minor is under the guardianship of the court of wards or a under a guardian appointed by court he is not deemed to attain his majority until he is 21 years age. A minor is incapable of selling his property and making a valid will to constitute an offence of kidnapping or abduction a minor from lawful guardianship the age of a boy should be under 16 years and that of a girl under 18 years.

Under the Factory Act 1848, an 'adult' is defined as a person who has completed his 18th year (an 'adolescent' is defined as a person who has completed his 15th but has not completed his 18th year). A "young person" means a person who is neither a child or an adolescent).

1

Medicolegal
Radiological
Age Determination

Chapter 1

Skeletal Anatomy

THE SKELETON

The skeleton in the living comprises long, short, small, flat and irregular bones having attachments of muscles, tendons, ligaments and cartilages. All these bones are covered by periosteum externally having elastic fibers, blood vessels and nerves. Long bones have proximal and distal ends expanded and articulate to form synovial joints. These ends are covered by articular cartilages and the joint space contains semilunar cartilages in some of the joints. Similarly the spinal column has vertebrae with bony projections and intervertebral disks in between two vertebrae. The shafts of long bones have marrow cavity filled with yellow bone marrow (fat/adipose tissue) and their expanded ends have red bone marrow hemopoietic). Long bones are tubular having thick compact bone. The middle part of the tubular shaft is thick and the expanded ends have trabecular bone covered by thin shell of compact bone. The ribs, vertebrae and the flat bones have spongy texture inside and have externally thin compact bone. Earlier, the long bones are rod-shaped cartilaginous models having similar shape of adult bones but are gradually converted into bony shafts in intrauterine life. At birth, these bony shafts have cartilaginous expanded ends in which secondary ossification centers are developed.

The primary ossification center develops in the central part of cartilaginous rod-shaped shaft and it spreads above and below to ossify the shaft. Most of the primary ossification centers are developed in eighth week of intrauterine life.

The proximal and distal cartilaginous ends ossify with multiple ossification centers after birth and thus they are transformed into bony ends. These secondary epiphyseal centers fuse (unite) with the diaphysis. The females show earlier ossification and epiphyseal "Fusion" than males. Most of the bones of the limbs have epiphyses at both ends and other short bones have it at one end only. At birth the proximal end of humerus is cartilaginous. Three secondary ossification centers are developed during childhood and unite together to form a single mass of composite epiphysis of proximal end of humerus and fuse with the diaphysis. Composite epiphyses occur at the proximal and distal ends of humerus and in the distal end of femur.

Ossification centers appear in distal end of femur and in the proximal end of Tibia immediately before birth.

Epiphyseal surface of diaphyseal end of shaft is nodular and has ridges in immature bones. The end is convex and the epiphysis forms a shallow cup over it. The epiphyseal end of diaphysis is the growing end of metaphysis.

Cartilaginous growth plate is placed between the epiphysis and the metaphysis. In a mature bone, the metaphyseal and epiphyseal ossification process encroach upon growth plate from either sides and no meeting bony fusion of epiphysis occurs, which is visualized as a dense epiphyseal line in radiograph. It is possible to divide radiologically the process of fusion of epiphysis with the diaphysis into four stages:

1. **Stage I:** "No union"– no evidence of commencement of union between epiphysis and diaphysis.
2. **Stage II:** "Partial union" – obliteration commences in the space between the epiphysis and the diaphysis.
3. **Stage III:** "Recent union" – space gets closed but the line of fusion is visible at the junction of epiphysis and diaphysis.
4. **Stage IV:** "Complete union" – epiphyseal space obliterated by bony fusion showing the same density as that of the shaft.

For elongation of bone chondrocytes in growth plate divide into longitudinal columns in long axis of the shaft and occupy the zone of cartilaginous growth plate. Epiphyseal plate growth is nearly equal at both ends, which gets ossified. Increase in lengths of bones in infancy and again at puberty is great.

The bones and cartilages are specialized connective tissues. They have collagen fibers and osteocyte cells embedded in an intercellular matrix, mineralize, and highly vascular having inorganic salts of calcium and phosphate. Organic matter in bones is mainly of collagen fibers.

Bone is formed by deposition of collagen fibers and salts of calcium and phosphate forming a mineralized matrix. They form concentric cylindrical arrangements around capillary blood vessels present inside Haversian canals in a mature bone.

Dense texture of living bone is from compact (ivory) bone with concentric cylindrical Haversian system with mineralized salts. The outer surface of living bones is covered by periosteum and the inner surface by the endosteum. These layers contain osteoblast cell, osteoclasts and other cells of bone formation, which help in modeling of bones. Osteoprogenitor cells are stromal cells, which give rise to formation of various other bone cells. Functionally osteoblast cells lay down bone and deposit minerals in bone matrix. Osteocytes are derived from osteoblasts. Osteoclasts are responsible for bone resorption. Live bones contain water, which gets reduced in old age and bone minerals increase.

Nutrient arteries enter the shafts of long bones obliquely through the nutrient foraminae and they divide into ascending and descending branches inside the medullary cavity and through the cortical capillaries and Haversian canals nutrition to the bone is supplied.

Most of the skull bones have intramembranous ossification. Initially mesenchymal cells multiply around network of capillaries and the ground substance with collagen fibers are laid subsequently. Osteoblasts cause calcification of the matrix from the deeper layer of the periosteum. The cranial bones ossify from many ossification centers.

Cartilages attached to the bones of skeleton are also of specialized tissue composed of fibers, cells and matrix. In intrauterine life the fetus has cartilaginous skeleton that is replaced by bone in shafts in eighth week of intrauterine life and after birth in cartilaginous proximal and distal ends. Blood supply of the cartilages is scanty. Hyaline cartilages are translucent and elastic. The costal, nasal, laryngeal and tracheobronchial cartilages are hyaline cartilages. These are prone to ossification.

Articular hyaline cartilages cover the articular ends of bone in synovial joints. White fibrocartilage consisting of white fibrous tissue bundles forms articular disks and is found in glenoid cavity of scapula and the acetabulum in hip bones. Yellow elastic cartilage is found in external ear and the epiglottis, which do not ossify. Bodies of vertebrae are trabecular inside and have thin cortical bone externally.

THE SKULL (FIGS 1.1A AND B)

The skull consists of 22 bones articulated to form the skeleton of head. It is divided into cranial vault and facial bones.

CRANIAL VAULT

It is mostly formed by the frontal and parietal bones and a small part posteriorly by the squamous part of occipital bone; having an outer table and an inner table of compact bone and in the middle a spongy layer (diploë) containing red marrow. It has coronal, sagittal and lambdoid sutures.

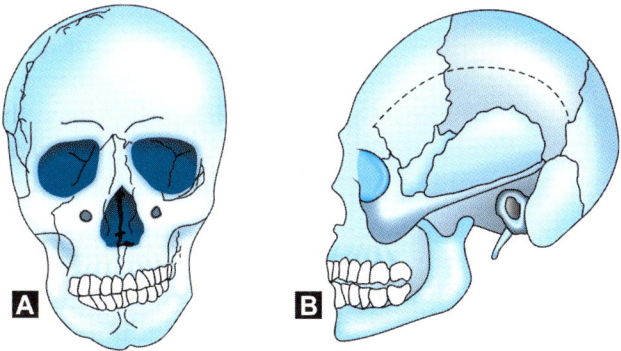

Figures 1.1A and B: (A) Skull (front view);
(B) Skull (lateral view)

The coronal suture is formed by joining serrated posterior border of frontal bone and the serrated anterior borders of two parietal bones.

The sagittal suture is formed in the median plane by the articulation of serrated sagittal borders of right and left parietal bones.

The lambdoid suture is formed by interlocking of more serrated lambdoid posterior borders of parietal bones with serrated lambdoid border of squamous part of occipital bone.

In each temporal fossa on the side of skull an H-shaped suture is formed by the articulation of frontal, parietal, temporal and greater wing of sphenoid bone with a small circular area around the center of the suture, which includes the four bones is the "pterion". The center of pterion is 4 cm above the zygomatic arch and 3.5 cm behind the frontozygomatic suture. The pterion marks internally the course of anterior branch of middle meningeal artery often injured in fissure fractures of skull in head injuries and cause epidural hemorrhage. Trephine hole is made by the neurosurgeon to remove the blood clot and ligate the blood vessel. Figure 1.2 shows schematic representation of CT scan image of cranium at the level of bodies lateral ventricles of brain.

Bones of Skull

Frontal bone forms the forehead of skull. It is less vertical and more steep in male than female. Frontal eminences are elevated areas of frontal bone of either side above the **superciliary arches** and are more prominent in female

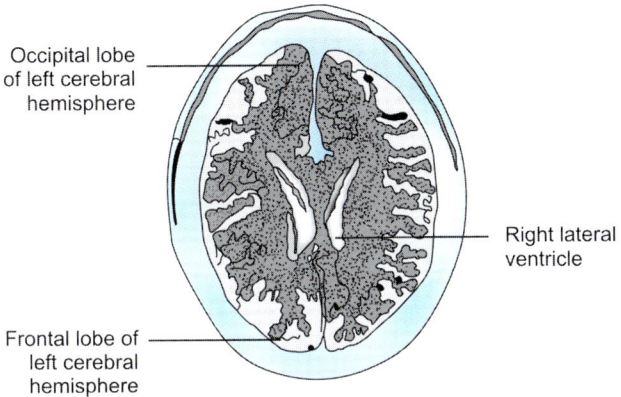

Figure 1.2: Schematic representation of CT scan image of cranium at the level of bodies lateral ventricles of brain

than in male. **Superciliary arches** are rounded bony elevations above the supraorbital margins of eye sockets in the frontal bone. These arches are more elevated in males. **Glabella** is a median bony elevation on forehead between the medial ends of superciliary arches, which is more marked in male. **Orbital openings** partly formed by frontal bones are nearly square shaped or quadrangular in male than in female.

In female, orbital openings are more rounded. One centimeter below the infraorbital margin is the infraorbital foramen through which infraorbital nerve and blood vessels emerge.

Frontal sinuses are asymmetrical irregular cavities situated lateral to the nasal spine and mostly deviated from the median plane. They are well developed in adult males than in females.

Parietal bones (paired) form part of cranial vault and sides of skull. They are nearly quadrilateral with convex external surface and with central parietal eminences. Internal surface of each parietal bone is concave and is marked by grooves of middle meningeal artery and vein.

Occipital bone (single): Occipital bone forms the posterior part of the skull and forms the part of base and vault. It comprises of three parts: squamous part, condylar part and Basilar part. The squamous part is posterior to foramen magnum. It is convex externally and concave internally. Outer surface has external occipital protuberance. The condylar parts are on either side of the foramen magnum. The basilar part extends forwards from foramen magnum and articulates anteriorly with the body of sphenoid.

Temporal bones (paired): Temporal bones are two. One on each side of skull and take part in formation of base of skull. Each temporal bone has squamous, petromastoid and tympanic parts. External temporal surface is slightly convex and its cerebral surface is concave. Its zygomatic processes extend forwards on each side from the lower part of squamous temporal bone and its serrated anterior end articulates with temporal process of zygomatic bone. In petromastoid parts, the mastoid part is the posterior region of temporal bone and projects down as mastoid process. Petrous part is a wedge between the sphenoid and occipital bones in the base of skull. Its apex contains the opening of carotid canal. The petrous part of temporal bone is of compact bone. Each styloid process projects from the lower aspect of temporal bone. It is pointed and about 2.5 cm in length.

Sphenoid bone (single): Sphenoid bone takes part in the formation of base of skull partly and is in between frontal, temporal and occipital bones. It comprises a body and two greater and two lesser wings. These wings spread laterally from lateral surface of the body. In front the body articulates with cribriform plate of ethmoid bone and posteriorly with basilar part of occipital bone by cartilage in between, which become bony after puberty. Dorsal aspect of the body has a pituitary fossa, which is concave. The body of sphenoid bone has two sinuses separated by a bony septum. Its greater wings fit on each side in the angle formed between the squamous part of temporal bone and the petrous bone. Lesser wings are triangular in shape.

Ethmoid bone (single): It is placed anteriorly in the base of skull with its cribriform plate. The perpendicular plate, which is flat, thin and quadrilateral is placed in median plane. It descends from inferior surface of cribriform plate to form the upper part of nasal septum.

Facial Bones

Maxillae (right and left) form the upper jaw and roof of the mouth. Thus they form the upper part of facial skeleton. The alveolar process of each maxilla is thick and arched and has sockets for the roots of upper teeth.

Maxillary sinus is a large cavity in each maxilla.

Zygomatic bones (paired) have convex lateral surface and form prominence of cheeks.

Palatine bones (paired) are L-shaped small bones, which form the posterior part of the hard palate; lateral walls of nasal cavity and part of posterior wall of orbit.

Lacrimal bones (paired) are small bones; one on either side and anteriorly placed in the medial wall of each orbital opening.

Vomer (single) is a thin and flat bone, which forms posteroinferior part of nasal septum.

Nasal bones (paired): These bones are small in size and are placed side by side. In the upper part they join with the frontal bone and form the nasal bridge. These nasal bones form upper border of the anterior nasal aperture, which is pear shaped; narrow above and wide below. Nasal aperture is bounded below by the maxillae.

Mandible: Mandible forms the lower part of facial skeleton. It has a curved body with its convexity externally and has two vertical and flat ramii.

Body of mandible has external and internal surfaces and upper and lower borders. Symphysis menti is formed in the midline by the fusion of two halves after fetal life. Symphysis menti is square shaped in male and in female it is uniformly curved.

Mental foramen is situated below and in line between the first and second premolar teeth or below the root of second premolar tooth. Mental nerve and mental blood vessels emerge through the mental foramen. The upper alveolar border contains roots of lower teeth. Mental foramen is central, i.e. midway between the upper and lower borders. In old age, it is nearer to the upper border due to alveolar absorption.

Ramus of the mandible is the ascending part of posterior end of the body of mandible, which is quadri-lateral and has condyloid and coronoid processes.

Coronoid process, which is thin and triangular, situated in its anterior part, and the condylar process, which is in posterior part articulates with temporal bone in the base of skull at the mandibular fossa. In early age groups the coronoid process in above the level of condylar process. **Angle of the mandible** is at the joining place of posterior and inferior border of lower jaw. It is everted in male and inverted in female. Mandibular foramen is situated little above the center on inner side of ramus overlapped on anteromedially by a triangular bony lingula. The mandibular foramen leads into the mandibular canal, which runs downwards and forwards in the body of mandible and opens externally into the mental foramen. **Myelohyoid canal** is located little above the myelohyoid line for the supply of alveolar nerves and blood vessels to the roots of lower teeth.

Myelohyoid line as a bony ridge on inner side of body of the mandible extending from behind the third molar tooth, obliquely lying 1 cm below the upper border of lower jaw at its commencement and extends obliquely on to the posterior side of symphysis menti. Myelohyoid groove descends forwards obliquely on inner surface of body of mandible commencing from behind the lingula and below the posterior part of myelohyoid line. The mandibular canal is nearly parallel to the myelohyoid line. The mandibular canal is nearly parallel to the myelohyoid line in adult and nearer to the upper border of mandible in old age.

Hyoid bone: Hyoid bone is situated in the anterior part of neck above the larynx and is at the joining place of front of neck and the floor of mouth. It is a U-shaped bone having a body and two greater cornua (two lesser cornua are insignificant). The greater cornua are connected to the body on either side by hyaline cartilage. In the living, the hyoid bone is suspended from tips of styloid processes of temporal bones by styloid ligaments having longer lengths. Body of hyoid bone is quadrilateral with convex anterior surface and concave posterior surface. In middle aged and in elderly individuals, the cartilage between the body and greater cornua is ossified into bone formation. When ossified the hyoid bone becomes a U-shaped bone. **Greater cornua** are flattened from above downwards and extend backwards from the lateral ends of body horizontally.

Larynx: Larynx is an airway lying opposite third to sixth cervical vertebrae in the anterior part of neck, below it is continuous with trachea. Thyroid cartilage, cricoid cartilage and epiglottis form cartilaginous skeleton of larynx.

Thyroid cartilage is more prominent in male and forms the Adam's Apple. It comprises of two quadrilateral laminae. Their anterior borders unite in their lower two-third and from laryngeal prominence. The posterior ends of thyroid cartilage project into superior and inferior cornua.

Cricoid cartilage form the lower part of larynx and is articulated above with the thyroid cartilage. Below, the cricoid cartilage is attached from its lower horizontal border to the trachea. Cricoid cartilage is like a signet ring having a narrow anterior arch and broad posterior lamina.

Epiglottis is a leaf-like fibrocartilage, which projects obliquely above and behind the hyoid bone.

Teeth: Deciduous (temporary) teeth are 20 in number and erupt from the sixth month to two years of childhood. Permanent teeth are 32. They replace temporary teeth from sixth year to 25 years.

Tooth consists of a crown, neck and root. The tooth is made of mostly dentine with enamel covering. The root is surrounded by alveolar bone. Grinding surfaces of crowns have cusps. Lower third molar tooth is smaller and has its roots fused. Third molar in lower jaw is often impacted against the second molar tooth. Third molar may be congenitally absent.

ERUPTION OF TEMPORARY TEETH

Central incisors	:	Sixth months
Lateral incisors	:	Seventh months
Canines	:	One and half year
First molar	:	First year
Second molar	:	Second year

ERUPTION OF PERMANENT TEETH

First molars	:	Sixth year
Central incisors	:	Seventh year
Lateral incisors	:	Eighth year
Canines	:	Eleventh year
First premolars	:	Ninth year
Second premolars	:	Tenth year
Second molars	:	Twelfth year
Third molars	:	Seventeen to twenty five years

THE VERTEBRAL COLUMN

The vertebral column consists of seven cervical, twelve thoracic and five lumbar vertebrae. Body of a vertebra is composed of cancellous trabecular bone internally and compact bone externally. Its transverse process on each side extends laterally from the joining site of pedicle and lamina. Pedicles are short and thick dorsal projections from upper part of the body of vertebra having notches on its upper and lower borders. Adjacent vertebral notches form intervertebral foramen. Laminae are bony plates continuous with pedicles on either side. Spinous processes are formed by uniting laminae in midline dorsally enclosing vertebral foramen. Articular processes (superior and inferior) extend from vertebral arch at union sites of pedicles and laminae.

INTERVERTEBRAL DISK (FIGS 1.3 AND 1.4)

Intervertebral disks are interposed between two vertebral bodies. They are of fibrocartilage. Each disk has an outer laminated annulus fibrosus and an inner nucleus pulposus. Annulus fibrosus has an outer collagenous zone and inner fibrocartilaginous zone. Nucleus pulposus is of fibrocartilage.

In cervical vertebrae, the spinous process is short and bifid. Superior surface of bodies of vertebrae are concave transversely with a prominent edge on each side. The anterior rim of inferior body surface of each vertebra projects downwards anterior to the inter-vertebral disk.

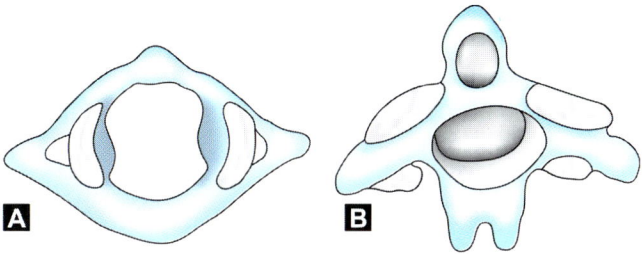

Figures 1.3A and B: (A) Atlas and (B) Axis

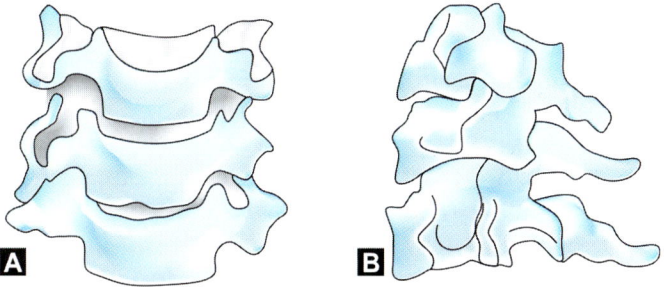

Figures 1.4A and B: 3rd, 4th and 5th cervical vertebrae
(Frontal and lateral view)

First cervical vertebra (Atlas): Comprises two lateral masses, an anterior arch and a posterior arch. It has no body and no spine.

Second cervical vertebra (Axis): Has an odontoid process, which projects from its upper surface. Pedicles of the vertebra have superior articular facets. Laminae are thick. Tip of spinous process is bifid.

Seventh cervical vertebra: Has a long spinous process, which is thick, horizontal and ends in a tubercle.

First thoracic vertebra resembles a cervical vertebra in shape. The spine is long, thick and horizontal. Other thoracic vertebrae have spinous process slanting backwards and downwards. The spinous process of eleventh thoracic vertebra is triangular and has horizontal lower border. The spinal cord occupies the vertebral canal and ends in lumbar region at the level of intervertebral disk between the first and second lumbar vertebra.

SACRUM AND COCCYX

Sacrum is a triangular bone formed by fusion of five sacral vertebrae. Dorsal surface of the sacrum is convex and the pelvic surface concave. Four transverse lines of fusion between vertebral bodies on pelvis surface are raised into bony ridges. In childhood individual, sacral vertebrae are connected by cartilage and gets separated on decomposition. The base of sacrum articulates with fifth lumbar vertebra and forms sacrovertebral angle. Sacral promontory is the anterior projecting edge of first sacral vertebral body and lateral parts of upper surface are ala of sacrum. A median sacral crest on dorsal aspects is formed by fusion of spines of sacral vertebrae. Pelvic surface of sacrum presents four pairs of pelvic sacral foramen. Lateral surface of sacrum on each side has an auricular surface, which articulates with ilium and forms fibrous articulation.

Coccyx is a small triangular bone, which articulates with the sacrum at its apex. It consists of four (three to five) rudimentary vertebrae. They reduce in size from upper to lower vertebrae.

In adult, the curvature of cervical vertebrae is convex forwards and extends from first cervical vertebra to the second thoracic vertebra. Thoracic curvature is concave forwards and extends from second to twelfth thoracic vertebra. Lumbar curve is convex forwards and extends from twelfth thoracic vertebra to the sacral angle. The pelvic curve is concave with sacrum and coccyx. It extends from lumbosacral junction to the apex of coccyx.

STERNUM (FIGS 1.5 TO 1.8)

The sternum is a long flat bone in the midline in front part of the thorax and is directed downloads and forwards. Its upper end articulates with the clavicles at sternoclavicular joints. Its lateral borders are attached to costal cartilages of seven upper pairs of ribs. The sternum is composed of cancellous bone covered by compact bone. It has three parts: Manubrium sterni, body and xiphisternum. Lower border of manubrium articulates with upper end of body of sternum and forms sternal angle. Body of sternum is long and narrow. It lies opposite at the level to fifth to

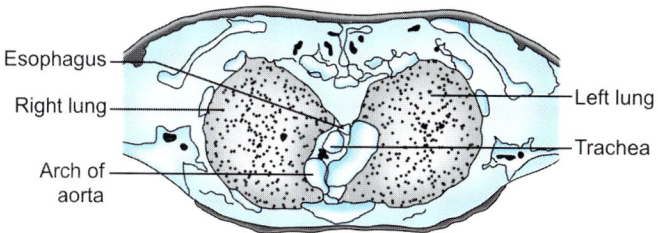

Figure 1.5: Schematic representation of CT scan at the level of the aortic arch

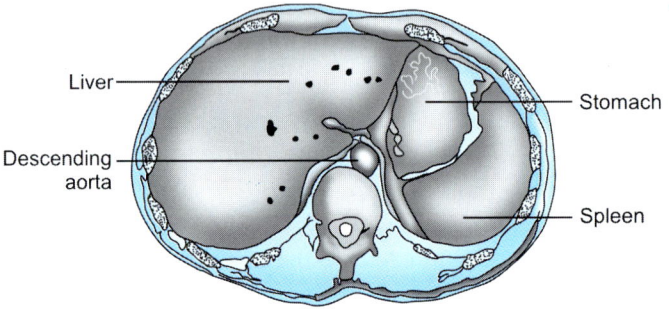

Figure 1.6: Schematic representation of CT scan of the abdomen at the level of esophageal opening of the diaphragm

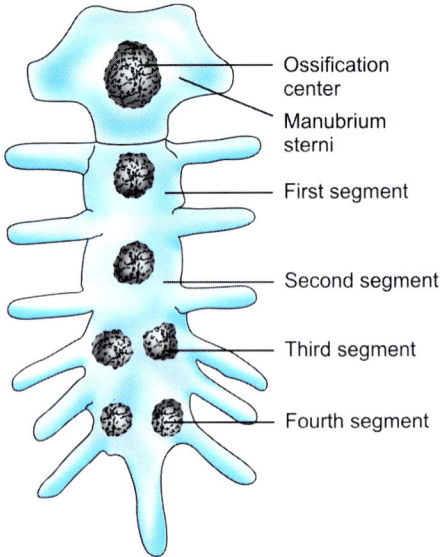

Figure 1.7: Ossification of sternum (before birth)

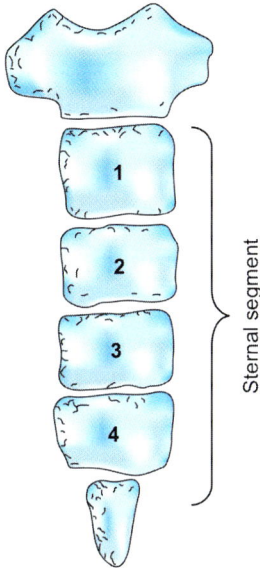

Figure 1.8: Ossification at 14 years (puberty)

ninth thoracic vertebra. At the fusion of four segments for sternum are marked by transverse ridges. Each lateral border has four notches of articulation of costal cartilages. Inferior border of body articulates with xiphisternum. Which lies in the epigastrium.

Ossification: One ossification center appears in manubrium sterni at 5th month of IUL, in first segment at 5th month IUL; in second and third segment (paired centers) in 6 to 7th month IUL and in fourth segment (paired centers) at 10th month IUL. All centers are present before birth. Ossification center of xiphoid process appears in 3 years. Manubrium sterni unites with the body in old age and the xiphisternum unites at 40 years of age.

RIBS

Ribs are composed of cancellous bone with the outer surface of compact bone. The ribs from 12 pairs of elastic arches and are connected posteriorly with the vertebral column. Anteriorly the upper seven pairs are connected by costal cartilages to the sternum. The lower five costal cartilages of eighth, nineth and tenth join to the adjacent upper cartilage, eleventh and twelfth ribs have free anterior ends (floating ribs).

COSTAL CARTILAGES

Costal cartilages are hyaline cartilages, which are flat and extend from the anterior ends of the ribs. Upper seven pairs join with the sternum and from the eighth to tenth join with the lower border of cartilage placed above. The lower two costal cartilages have free pointed ends.

CLAVICLES (FIG. 1.9)

Clavicles extend laterally and are placed horizontal across the anterior part of neck extending from manubrium sterni to the acromion. They are subcutaneous and prominent. The shaft is convex forwards in its medial two-thirds and concave forwards in its lateral one-third. Sternal end of each clavicle articulates with manubrium sterni at the clavicular notch and the joint has a fibrocartilaginous disk between the sternal end and the clavicular notch.

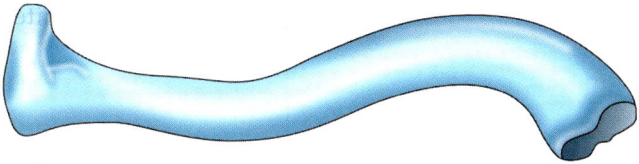

Figure 1.9: Clavicle/collar bone

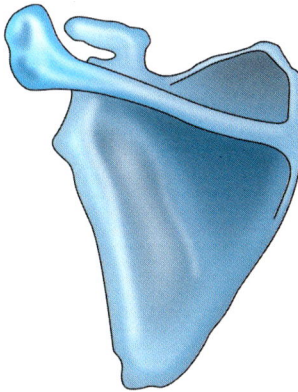

Figure 1.10: Scapula

Ossification: Two primary ossification centers appear and develop in the shaft in five weeks IUL and one secondary center for the sternal end of clavicle appears in 14 years and fuses at 20-22 years.

SCAPULA (FIG. 1.10)

Scapula is a large, flat and triangular bone having a thick lateral border. Inferior angle of scapula overlies the seventh rib or the seventh intercostal space in the living. Glenoid cavity is situated in its lateral angle and on articulation with head (proximal end) of humerus forms the shoulder joint. The spine of scapula projects from its dorsal surface. Acromion process projects forwards at right angle from the lateral end of spine and is subcutaneous. Coracoid process arises from the head of scapula and hooks laterally and forwards. Coracoacromion articulation forms an arch over the shoulder joint. Acromioclavicular joint is formed between the clavicle and the medial margin of the acromion.

Ossification: One primary ossification center appears in the body in 8th week of IUL. Two secondary centers for the coracoid process, one for the acromion process, two for the glenoid cavity; one for the inferior angle of scapula and one center for the vertebral border. The secondary ossification center for the coracoid process appears at one year and for the root at 10-11 years. Centers of coracoid process fuse at 15-16 years.

The secondary center of acromion fuses at 17-18 years; of glenoid cavity at 14-15 years; inferior angle of scapula at 17-18 years and of vertebral border at 14-15 years.

HUMERUS (FIGS 1.11A AND B)

Humerus is the long bone of upper arm having shaft, proximal and distal ends. The proximal rounded hemisphere forms the shoulder joint by articulating with the glenoid cavity of scapula. The head has greater and lesser tuberosities with a sulcus between them. The shaft is cylindrical with a narrow cavity and is of compact bone. Distal end is divided into capitulum, trochlea, medial and lateral condyles. It has a large olecranon fossa and coronoid and radial small fossae.

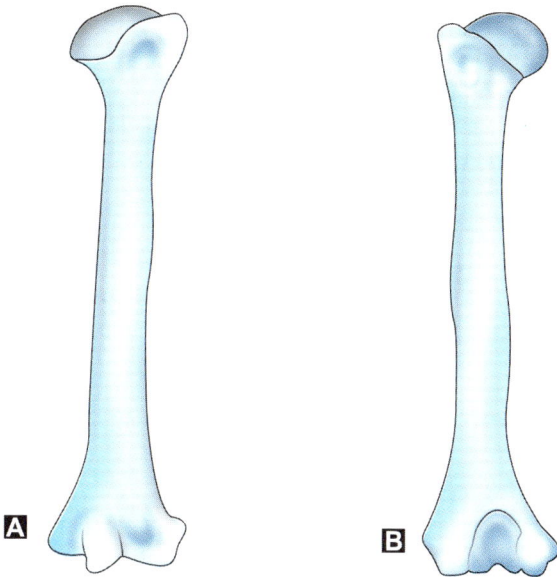

Figures 1.11A and B: Humerus (A) anterior aspect;
(B) posterior aspect

Capitulum is rounded and hemispherical, which
articulates with the head of radius in its shallow
depression. Trochlea is pully-like and articulates with the
trochlear notch of ulna. Medial epicondyle is a prominent
projection from its medial side and lateral epicondyle is
on lateral side forming the end of lateral border of
humerus. Olecranon fossa is a deep depression on the
posterior surface of lower end of humerus proximal to the
trochlea in which the apex of the olecranon fits in.

Ossification: One primary ossification center appears in the
middle of shaft in 8th week of IUL and three secondary
centers in the head (for head in 1 year; in greater tuberosity
in 3 years and in lesser tuberosity in 5 years). Four

secondary ossification centers appear in the lower end; (for capitulum in one year; in medial epicondyle 5-7 years; for trochlea 9-11 years; and in lateral epicondyle 11 years). Secondary centers fuse to shaft in proximal end at 18 years and in distal end from 14 to 16 years.

ELBOW JOINT (FIGS 1.12A AND B)

The elbow joint is the articulation between trochlea of lower end of humerus and ulnar trochlear notch and between capitulum of lower end of humerus and the head of radius.

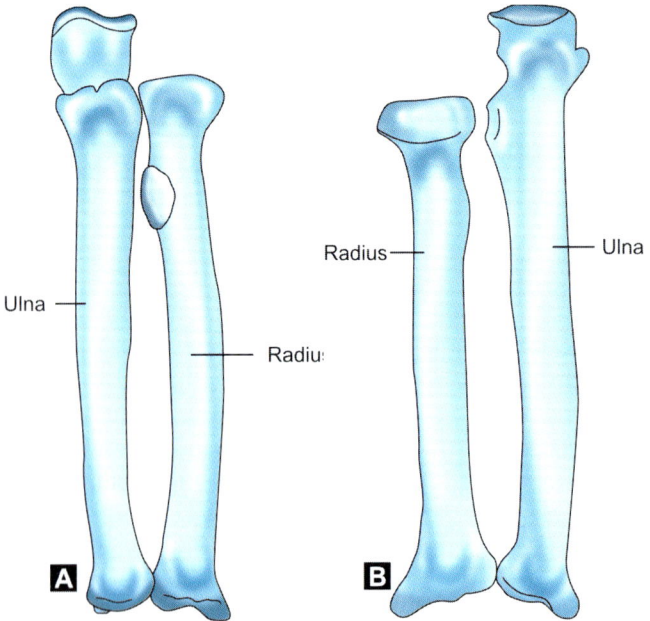

Figures 1.12A and B: Radius and ulna (A) anterior aspect (B) posterior aspect

RADIUS

Radius is placed on lateral side in the forearm. It has a proximal end forming head of radius with a shallow surface for the articulation with capitulum. The shaft has lateral convexity. The distal end of radius is expanded and projects as the styloid process distally.

Ossification: Primary ossification center appear in shaft in eighth week of IUL. Secondary ossification center appears in head in 5 years and fuses at 16 years. The secondary center, which appears in lower end in 2 years fuses at 18 years.

ULNA

Ulna is placed medial to the radius in the forearm. The proximal end is hook-like and concave forwards. The distal end has a styloid process. Proximal end has olecranon and coronoid processes; trochlear and radial notches for articulation with distal end of humerus and proximal end of radius. Trochlear notch of ulna articulates with trochlea of humerus at the distal end and forms the elbow joint.

Ossification: Primary ossification center appears for shaft in eighth week of IUL. Secondary ossification center appears in olecranon at 9th year and fuses at 16th year; and secondary center in lower end, which appears in 5-6 years fuses at 18 years.

THE WRIST JOINT AND THE HAND

WRIST JOINT

The wrist joint is formed by articulation of distal end of radius; scaphoid; lunate; triquetral and distal end of ulna.

The wrist contains eight carpal bones forming a proximal and a distal row. In the proximal row, the carpal bones placed from lateral to medial side are: scaphoid, lunate, triquetral, and pisiform. In the distal row from lateral to medial side are: trapezium, trapezoid, capitate and hamate. The pisiform articulates with the palmar surface of triquetral.

Ossification: Carpal bones are cartilaginous in fetal life and they ossify to become bony only after birth. Each cartilaginous carpal ossifies with one ossification center but at different periods. Ossification center in the capitate appears in 2 months, in hamate 3 months; in triquetral in 3 years; in lunate in 4 years; in trapezium 4-5 years; in trapezoid 4-5 years; in scaphoid in 4-5 years and in pisiform in 10-12 years.

METACARPAL BONES

They are five in number and are placed from lateral to the medial side. They are long bones having smaller lengths. Each metacarpal is having a distal end as head; middle part as shaft; and the base which is an expanded end. The rounded heads of metacarpals articulate with the phalanges and the bases articulate with the carpal bones. The first metacarpal bone is short and thick and its base articulates with the trapezium. The second metacarpal bone has a long shaft and the large base. The third metacarpal bone has a styloid process projecting from the radial side of base which articulates with the capitate. The fourth metacarpal bone is short and thin. Its base is in contact with the capitate and hamate. Fifth metacarpal bone has a tubercle on medial side of its base and the base articulates with the hamate.

Ossification: The shafts of five metacarpal bones develop their primary ossification centers in 9th week of IUL. The secondary ossification center for the base of first metacarpal bone appears in 2-3 years and unites with shaft in 15-17 years. Metacarpal heads of other four metacarpals ossify at 1.5-2.5 years and unite to their shafts at 15-19 years.

PHALANGES OF HAND AND FINGERS

The thumb has two phalanges and the other four fingers have three phalanges in each finger. Thus, fourteen phalanges are in the hand and its fingers. Each phalanx has a head, a shaft; and a proximal base. Shafts of all phalanges are tapering distally. The heads of middle and proximal phalanges are pully-like.

The shafts of proximal row of phalanges develop primary ossification center in 10th week; for middle row in 12 weeks and in terminal row in 8 weeks IUL. The secondary ossification centers of bases of phalanges appear at 2-4 years and fuse at 15-18 years.

PELVIS

Right and left hip bones articulate with the sacrum on either side and form the pelvis.

HIP BONES (FIGS 1.13A AND B)

Hip-bones are large irregular bones having a cup-shaped deep acetabulum on their lateral side and obturator foramen in their lower parts.

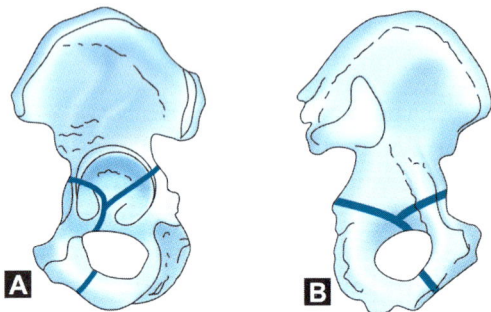

Figures 1.13A and B: Hip bone
(A) outer aspect (B) inner aspect

Each hip bone has three parts: ilium, ischium and pubis united by the triradiate cartilage in younger age group and becomes bony in adults. Ilium presents expanded appearance. Iliac crest is the upper border of ilium, which is convex and has internal and external lips. Its posterior border joining with posterior ischial border forms the greater sciatic notch. Auricular surface is "L" shaped, which articulates with sacrum and forms sacroiliac joint. A preauricular sulcus is present in female than in male. Pubis is the part of hip bone, which takes part in forming the pubic symphysis. The pubis has a superior ramus and an inferior ramus.

Ossification: Primary ossification center for ilium appears at about 8th week IUL; for ischium at about 12th week IUL and for pubis at about 18th week IUL. Secondary ossification center appears for the crest of ilium in 14 years and fuses at 20 years; in triradiate cartilage (acetabulum) 13 years and fuse at 13 to 15, in pubis appears at 14 years and fuse at 20 years, and in ischium appears at 16 years and fuse at 20-21 years.

HIP JOINT

The head of femur articulates with acetabulum and has ligaments and fibrous joint capsule. A fibrocartilaginous rim is attached to the margin of acetabulum. A flat band of ligament is attached from the sides of acetabular notch to the pit on head of femur.

FEMUR (FIGS 1.14A AND B)

Femur is the longest and strongest bone of all the long bones of skeleton. The shaft is cylindrical and convex anteriorly. The proximal end of femur consists of head, neck, greater trochanter and lesser trochanter. It has intertrochanteric line anteriorly and intertrochanteric crest posteriorly.

The head has articular surface little more than half of the sphere, which articulates in the acetabulum to form the hip joint. The neck of femur is 5 cm long forming an angle of about 125°. Intertrochanteric line is marked on the anterior surface at the junction of the neck and shaft and on posterior surface intertrochanteric crest. The greater trochanter is quadrangular and projects upwards from the junction of the neck and shaft. On its medial surface the greater trochanter has trochanteric fossa. Lesser trochanter is a conical projection on posteromedial aspect of the junction. The shaft is convex anteriorly and cylindrical in shape having medullary cavity filled with yellow bone marrow. The proximal and distal ends of femur have trabecular bone filled with the red bone marrow and have outer shell of compact bone. The distal end is expanded and has two large condyles having

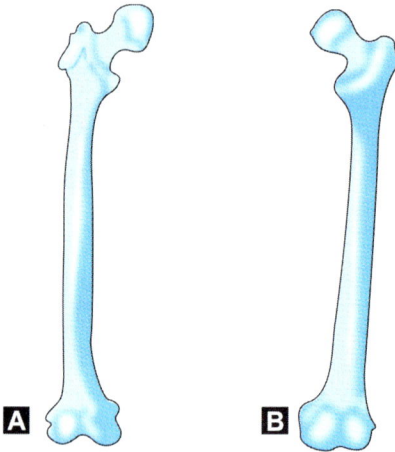

Figures 1.14A and B: Femur
(A) anterior aspect (B) posterior aspect

articular surfaces and intercondylar fossa. The patella is placed anterior to both condyles. Lateral condyle at the lower end of femur is flat laterally and less prominent on the medial side. It is directly in the line of femoral shaft and lateral epicondyle is the prominent point on the lateral condyle.

Medial condyle is convex and bulges on its medial side. Its medial side has medial epicondyle.

Ossification: One primary ossification center appears in the shaft in eight week IUL. Secondary center appears in head in 0.5-1 year; in greater trochanter in 4 years; lesser trochanter in 12-14 years; and in the lower end of femur in 9 months IUL or at birth and they unite to the shaft at 18 years.

KNEE JOINT

Knee joint is a large joint formed by articulation of distal end of femur and proximal end of tibia (and the patella placed anteriorly) with cartilaginous meniscii and strong ligaments inside the joint. The condyles of the femur articulate with tibial articular surfaces on medial and lateral condyles. Line diagram showing the MRI image of knee joint in sagittal section is shown in Figure 1.15.

PATELLA

Patella is the largest sesamoid bone embedded in the tendon of quadriceps femoris muscle and is placed anterior to the knee joint. Its anterior surface is convex and in the living the surface is subcutaneous. The posterior surface has a large articular lateral facet, which is in contact

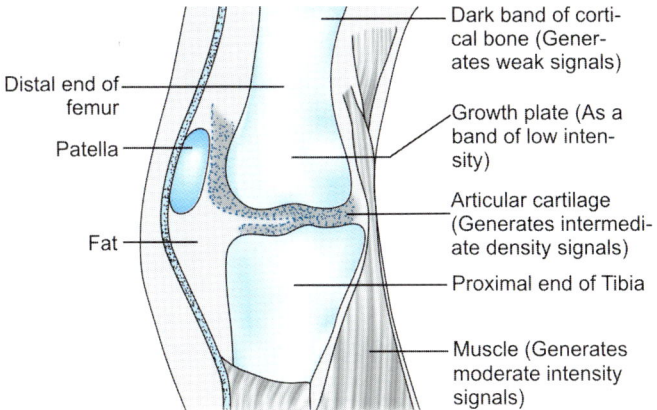

Figure 1.15: Line drawing of MRI image of the knee joint (sagittal section medial to the head of fibula)

with the medial femoral condyle. A vertical ridge divide the lateral facet with the medial facet. Patella is triangular distally and forms "APEX", which gives attachment to patellar ligament. The patella consists of trabecular bone and is covered by thick compact bone.

Ossification: 3 years.

TIBIA (FIGS 1.16A AND B)

The proximal end of tibia has medial and lateral condyles having articular surfaces. Medial articular surface is oval and lateral articular surface circular and they are slightly concave to fit the femoral condyles. The intercondylar area has raised medial and lateral intercondylar tubercles. The shaft is triangular. The proximal and distal ends of tibia

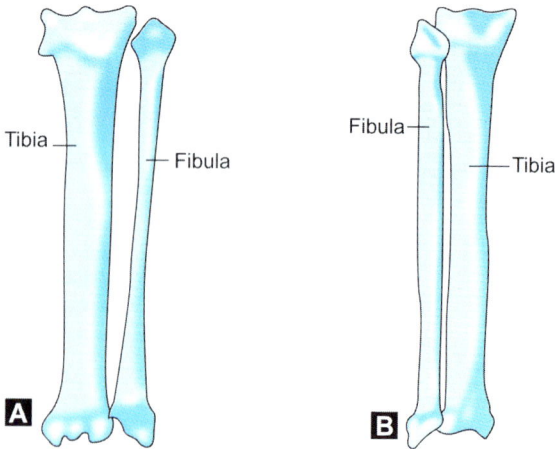

Figures 1.16A and B: Tibia and fibula (A) anterior aspect (B) posterior aspect

are expanded. The distal end projects downwards on medial side as the medial malleolus. The distal surface of lower end of tibia articulates with talus.

Ossification: One primary ossification center appears in the shaft in eighth week of IUL. A secondary ossification center appears in the proximal end of tibia at birth or 9 months of IUL and unites at 18th year. The secondary ossification center, which appears in the lower end in 1 year and fuses to shaft at 16th year.

FIBULA

Fibula is a thin bone. It has a head, shaft and distal malleolus. Head is the proximal expanded end of the bone. Distal end forms the lateral malleolus.

Ossification: Primary center for the shaft appears at eighth week IUL. A secondary center for proximal end appears at 4 years and unites at 18th year. At distal end center appears at 1 year and unites at 16th year.

ANKLE AND FOOT (FIG. 1.17)

Ankle and foot have tarsal bones, metatarsal bones and phalanges. The tarsal bones are seven in number and form the skeleton of proximal half of the foot by forming proximal and distal rows. Calceneum and talus form the proximal row. The three cuneiform bones, i.e. medial, intermediate and lateral cuneiform and the cuboid form the distal row. The navicular bone is placed between the talus and the cuneiform bones. The tarsal bones are composed of cancellous bone. Talus takes part in the

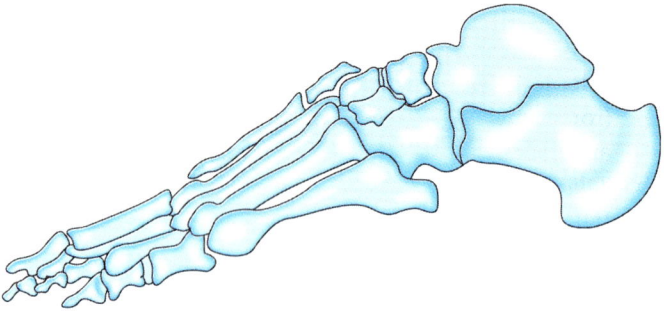

Figure 1.17: Foot bones (lateral view)

formation of ankle joint with its trochlear surface with the distal end of tibia. The head of talus articulates with proximal surface of navicular bone. The plantar surface of head of talus articulates on medial projection of calceneum. The navicular bone articulates proximally with head of talus and distally with three cuneiform bones. The cuneiform bones articulate proximally with navicular bone and bases of first to third metatarsal bones distally. The cuboid is placed proximally between calceneum and distally to the fourth and fifth metatarsals.

ANKLE JOINT

The ankle joint is formed by the lower end of tibia, medial malleolus of tibia; lateral malleolus of fibula and trochlear surface of talus.

METATARSAL BONES

Five metatarsal bones are placed distal in the foot articulating with tarsals proximally with their bases and with phalanges distally with their heads.

Ossification of ankle and foot bones

a. *Calcaneum:* The primary ossification center appears in calcaneum in 5th month IUL and its secondary center (for posterior part) of calcaneum appears at 6-8 years and fuses at 14-16 years.

b. *Talus:* Talus primary ossification appears at 7 month of IUL.

c. *Navicular:* Ossification center appears in 3 years.

d. *Cuboid:* Ossification center appears in 9 months of IUL/ at birth.

Cuneiform bones

a. *Medial cuneiform:* Ossification center appears in 2 years.

b. *Middle cuneiform:* Ossification center appears in third year.

c. *Lateral cuneiform:* Ossification center appears in 1 year.

First Metatarsal Bone

The primary ossification center appears in 10 weeks and the secondary ossification center for the base appears in 3 years and unites at 17-20 years.

Second Metatarsal Bone

The primary ossification center appears in 9 weeks IUL (and also for third, fourth and fifth metatarsal bones) and the secondary ossification center for heads appears in 3-4 years. The heads of second to fifth metatarsal bones unite to their shafts in 17-20 years.

PHALANGES

The primary ossification center for shafts appear in 11-15 weeks IUL for the first row and secondary ossification centers for their bases appear in 2-8 years. The bases of phalanges unite at the age of 18 years. For the middle phalanges, the primary ossification center appears in 15 weeks of IUL and secondary centers in 3-6 years. The bases unite to their shafts in 18 years. The primary ossification centers for the shafts of terminal phalanges appear in 9-12 weeks IUL and secondary center for their bases appear in 6 years. The bases of distal phalanges unite to their shafts in 18 years.

Chapter 2

Lower Jaw for Development of the Third Molar Tooth

Radiograph of lower jaw lateral view shows: Third molar tooth has erupted completely. Grinding surfaces of teeth are not showing any attrition (Figs 2.1 to 2.3).

Opinion: As per the radiological examination the age of the individual is of adult (above 25 years and below 35 years)

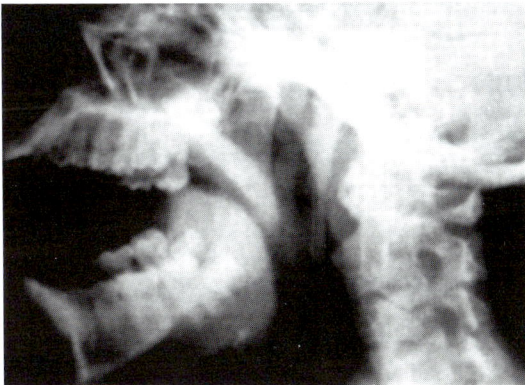

Figure 2.1: Erupting third molar tooth in the stage of crown formation (lateral view radiograph of lower jaw)

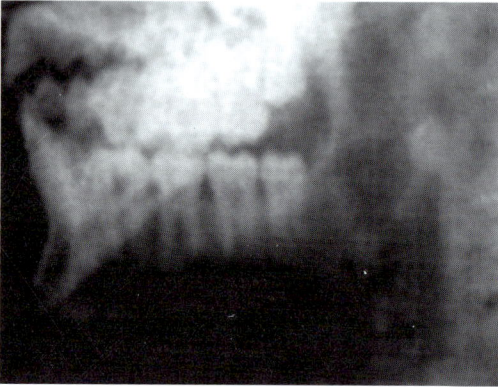

Figure 2.2A: X-ray of lower jaw—lateral view

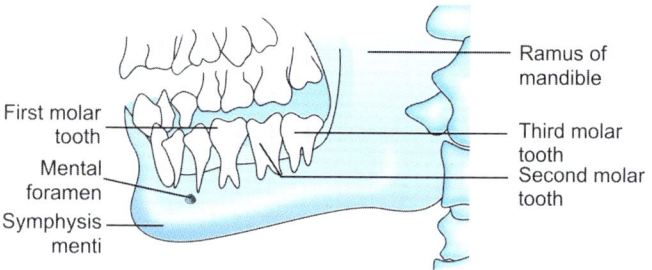

Figure 2.2B: Outline of lateral radiograph of lower jaw (mandible)

OTHER IMPORTANT POINTS

- Up to the age 25 years and after fetal life, dentition and ossification provides assessment of age with accuracy.
- Teeth are radiopaque and the pulp of teeth is radiolucent.

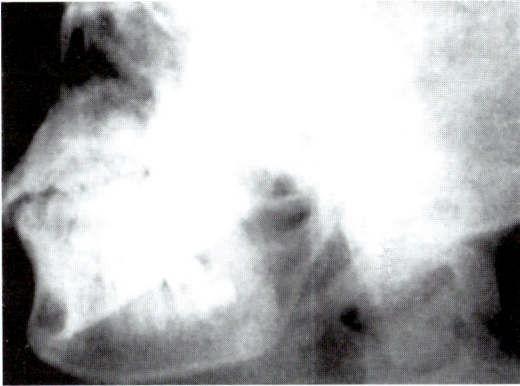

Figure 2.3A: X-ray of lower jaw—lateral view

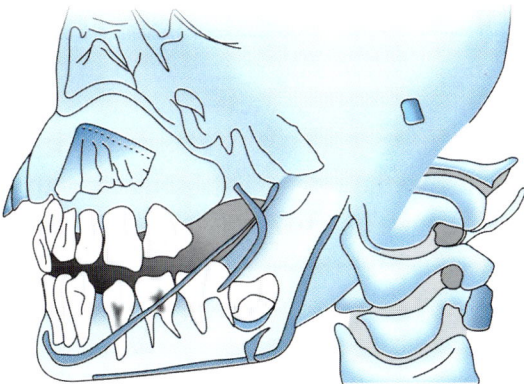

Figure 2.3B: Outline of lateral radiograph of lower jaw
(Mandible)

Third molar tooth shows only crown formation inside the alveolar bone of lower jaw. The space is formed behind the second molar tooth.

Opinion: As per the radiological examination, the age of the individual is above 12 years and below 14 years [i.e. about 12-13 years].

OTHER IMPORTANT POINTS
• Hyoid bone is situated at the meeting place of front of the neck and the floor of the mouth. • Mylohyoid line gives attachment to the mylohyoid muscle on the inner side of body of mandible. • The mentum is projecting and square-shaped; it reveals the male sex.

Lateral Radiograph of lower jaw and the neck shows: Third molar tooth in its root formation. The crown is formed and impinging against the second molar tooth. Body of hyoid bone on either side is not united to the greater cornuae indicating the presence of cartilaginous joints (Figs 2.4A and B).

Opinion: As per the radiological examination, the age of the individual is about 15 years.

OTHER IMPORTANT POINTS
• The location of first and second premolar teeth is possible in lower jaw from the site of mental foramen as it is located normally below the root of second premolar tooth. • In adult the grinding surfaces of teeth do not show any attrition. It occurs in advanced age due to wear and tear from mastication. • Coronoid process of mandible is triangular flattened projection in anterior part of mandibular notch, which is a depression between coronoid and condyloid process.

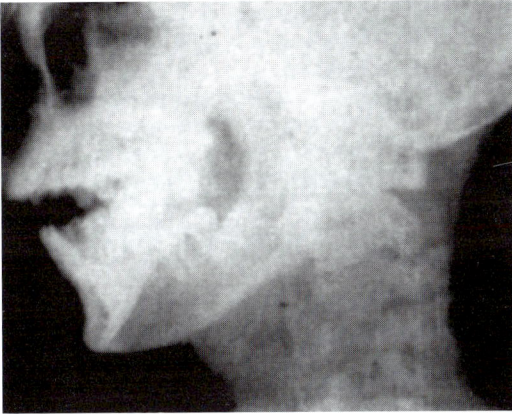

Figure 2.4A: X-ray of lower jaw and the neck—lateral view

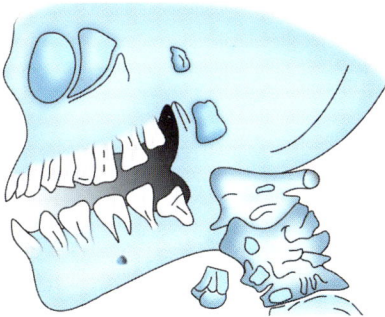

Figure 2.4B: Outline of lateral radiograph of lower jaw and the neck

Lateral radiograph of lower jaw shows: Third molar tooth developed completely but 'impacted'. The third molar is making an angle with the second molar tooth and its crown impinges against the second molar tooth. Grinding surfaces of teeth do not show any attrition (Figs 2.5A and B).

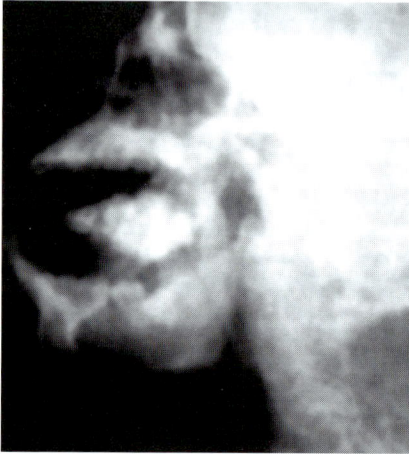

Figure 2.5A: X-ray of lower jaw—lateral view

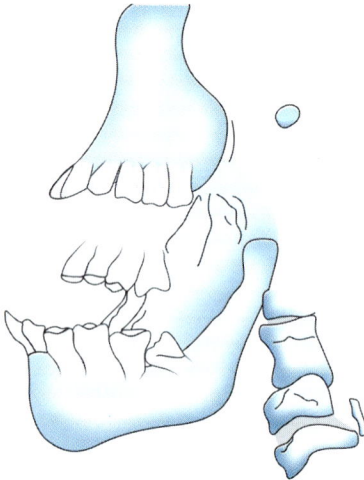

Figure 2.5B: Outline of lateral radiograph of lower jaw

Opinion: As per the radiological examination, the age of the individual is of adult (above 21 years and below 30 years).

Radiograph of lower jaw lateral view (Figs 2.6A and B) shows

- Congenital absence of third molar tooth in the lower jaw.
- Grinding surfaces of teeth do not show any attrition.

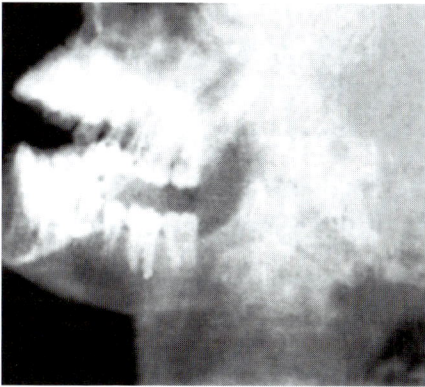

Figure 2.6A: X-ray of lower jaw—lateral view

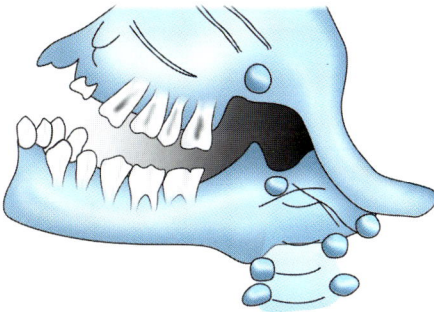

Figure 2.6B: Outline of lateral radiograph of lower jaw

Opinion: As per the radiological examination, the age is of adult (below 35 years and above 12 years).

OTHER IMPORTANT POINTS
• Tooth germs are formed in alveolar bone in third or fourth month IUL, crown is formed first.
• At birth complete development of the crown is seen with rudimentary root formation.
• During eruption of permanent teeth the roots of temporary teeth undergo absorption and their crowns fall off.
• Canine tooth is longer, has a conical crown and produces bulge externally, i.e. canine eminence in alveolar margins of both jaws.

Chapter 3

Shoulder Joint

■■■■■■■■■■■■■■■■■■■■■■■■

COLLAR BONE AND SHOULDER JOINT (FIG. 3.1)

COLLAR BONE

Ossification centers {appearance (A) and fusion (F)}:
1. Primary center
   Shaft: 4-5 weeks (A) IUL
2. Secondary center
   Inner end: 15-19 years (A), 20-22 years (F)

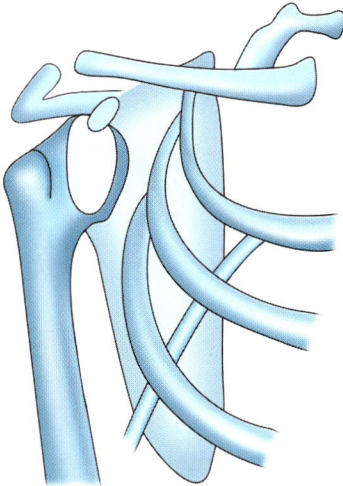

Figure 3.1: Right collar bone and right shoulder joint

SHOULDER JOINT

1. **Primary ossification center:** For shaft of humerus, 8 weeks IUL.
2. **Secondary ossification centers:** For proximal end of humerus
   - Head: 1 year (A)
   - Greater tuberosity: 3 years (A)
   - Lesser tuberosity: 5 years (A)
     Head of humerus and tuberosities 5-6 years (F) and form a conjoint epiphysis, and the conjoint epiphysis unites with the shaft at 18-19 years (F).

SCAPULA

PRIMARY OSSIFICATION CENTER FOR BODY OF SCAPULA

8 weeks IUL

SECONDARY OSSIFICATION CENTERS

- Glenoid cavity   : 14-15 years (A), 17 years (F).
- Acromion process   : 14-15 years (A), 17-18 years (F).
- Coracoid process (tip) : 10-11 years (A), 16 years (F)

Radiograph of left shoulder joint AP view shows (Figs 3.2 and 3.3)

- Epiphysis of proximal end of humerus: Fused and shows epiphyseal line.
- Epiphysis of acromion process: Fused.

Opinion: As per the radiological examination of left shoulder.
The age of the individual is about 21 years.

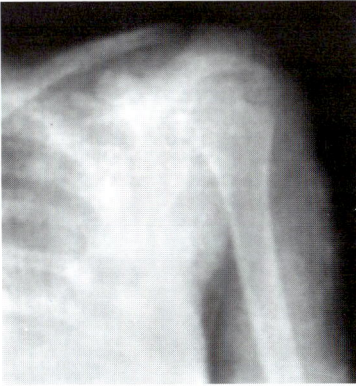

Figure 3.2: Anteroposterior view of left shoulder joint
(showing scapula)

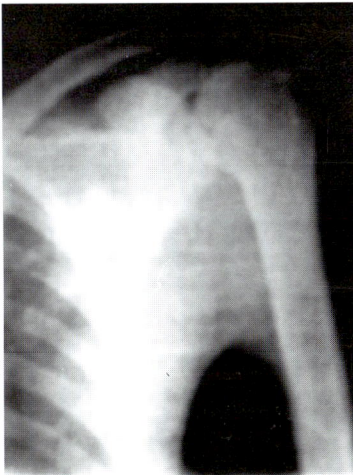

Figure 3.3A: X-ray of left shoulder joint AP view

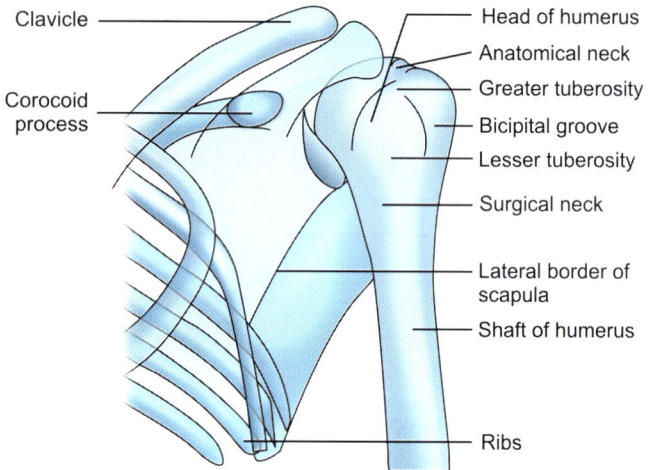

Figure 3.3B: Outline of radiograph anteroposterior view of left shoulder

OTHER IMPORTANT POINTS

- The process of fusion in the proximal end of humerus is nearly complete but the epiphyseal line can be distinguished.
- Epiphyseal line does not indicate recent union.
- Bicipital groove is the intertubercular groove present between the greater and lesser tubercle of humerus.
- Acromion process is seen forming a sort of hood above the shoulder joint.
- The proximal end of the humerus is cartilaginous at birth. In childhood, three separate secondary centers are developed in the cartilaginous end.
- When all the epiphyses of bones of the skeleton are united. It is possible to estimate the age of the individual as above 25 years.

Radiograph of right shoulder shows (Figs 3.4A and B)

- Epiphysis of head of humerus and greater tuberosity: Fused.
- Epiphysis of proximal end of humerus not fused with the shaft.

Opinion: As per the radiological examination, the age of the individual is above 6 years and below 18 years.

OTHER IMPORTANT POINTS

- Epiphyseal plate is the binding cartilage between the epiphysis and the diaphysis, which is radiolucent in radiograph.
- Secondary ossification centers of head, greater tuberosity and lesser tuberosity fuse together and form a single epiphysis, which later fuses to the diaphysis.

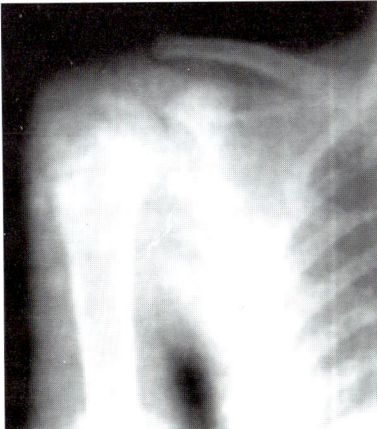

Figure 3.4A: X-ray of right shoulder—AP view

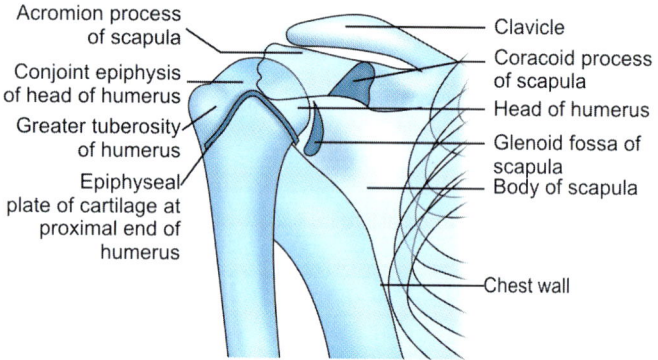

Figure 3.4B: Outline of AP radiograph of right shoulder

Radiograph of right shoulder AP view shows: Epiphysis of acromion process appeared and not fused (Figs 3.5A and B).

Opinion: As per the radiological examination, the age is above 14 years and below 18 years.

OTHER IMPORTANT POINT
Conjoint epiphysis of head of humerus is formed by union of epiphysis of head and greater tuberosity at the age of 6 years.

AP radiograph of left shoulder shows: Conjoint epiphysis of proximal and of humerus not formed. Epiphyses of acromion process not appeared (Figs 3.6A and B).

Opinion: The age of the individual as per the radiological examination is above 5 years and below 6 years (epiphysis of head of humerus and epiphysis of greater tuberosity not united).

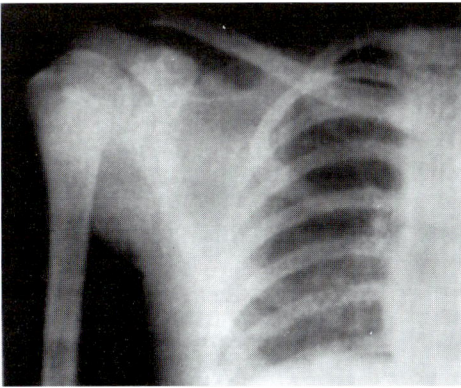

Figure 3.5A: X-ray of right shoulder—AP view

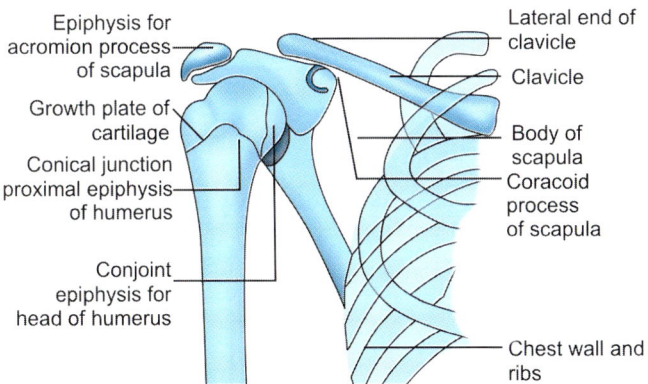

Figure 3.5B: Outline of AP view radiograph of right shoulder

OTHER IMPORTANT POINTS

- The proximal end of humerus shows "no union" of epiphysis with the shaft.
- Epiphysis of head of humerus and greater tuberosity unites at about 6 years and forms conjoint epiphysis.

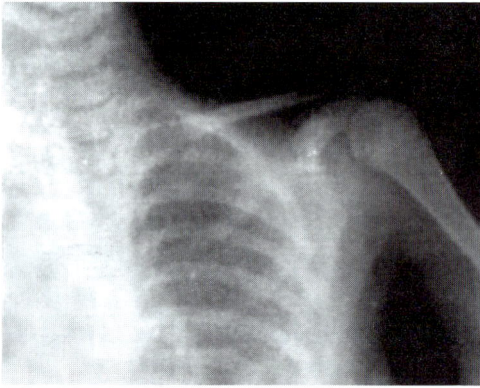

Figure 3.6A: X-ray of left shoulder—AP view

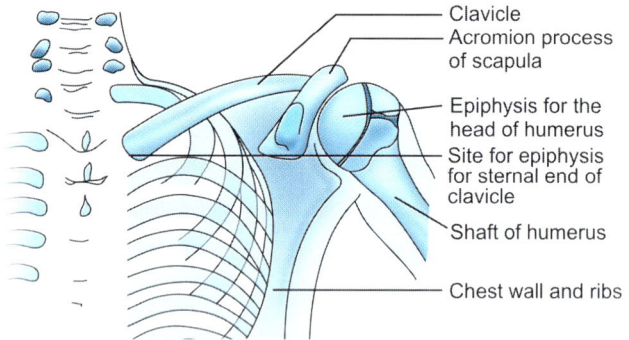

Figure 3.6B: Outline of AP view radiograph of left shoulder

AP radiograph of left shoulder shows: Epiphysis of head of humerus; greater tuberosity and lesser tuberosity not united to form conjoint epiphysis of proximal end of humerus. Epiphyses of proximal end are not united to the shaft (Figs 3.7A and B).

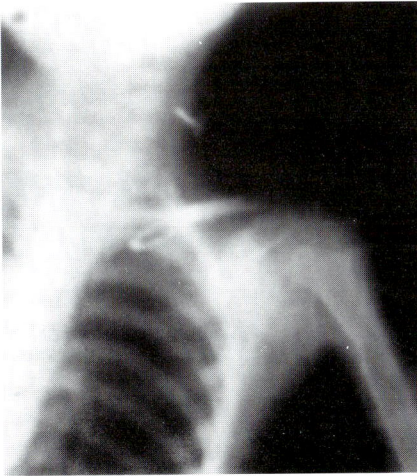

Figure 3.7A: X-ray of left shoulder—AP view

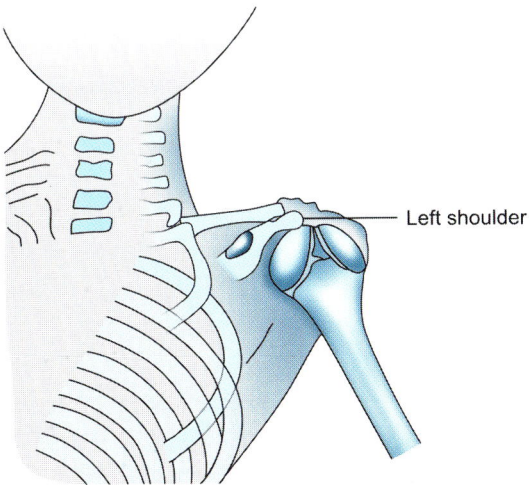

Left shoulder

Figure 3.7B: Outline of AP radiograph of left shoulder

Opinion: The age of individual as per the radiological examination is above 3 years and below 5 years (epiphysis of greater tuberosity appeared and lesser tuberosity did not appear).

OTHER IMPORTANT POINTS

- Primary ossification centers appear in eight week IUL.
- At the proximal end of humerus ossification centers of head; greater tuberosity and lesser tuberosity join at about sixth year and form a large epiphysis.

Chapter 4

Elbow Joint

HUMERUS (FIG 4.1)

PRIMARY OSSIFICATION CENTER

- For shaft of humerus:
  - 8 weeks (IUL)

SECONDARY OSSIFICATION CENTER AT DISTAL END

(Distal end of humerus)
- Capitulum:
  - 1 year (A)
  - 14-16 years (F)

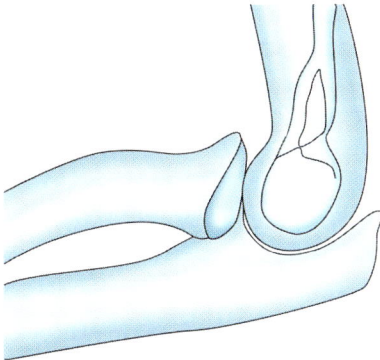

Figure 4.1: Elbow joint

- Medial epicondyle:
  - — 5-7 years (A)
  - — 14-16 years (F)
- Lateral epicondyle:
  - — 11 years (A)
  - — 14-16 years (F)
- Trochlea:
  - — 9-11 years (A)
  - — 14-16 years (F).

RADIUS

PRIMARY OSSIFICATION CENTER

- For shaft of radius:
  - — 8 weeks IUL

SECONDARY OSSIFICATION CENTERS AT DISTAL END

- For head of radius:
  - — 5 years (A)
  - — 16-17 years (F)
- For lower end of radius:
  - — 2 years (A)
  - — 18 to 19 years (F).

ULNA

PRIMARY OSSIFICATION CENTER

- For shaft of ulna:
  - — 8 weeks IUL

SECONDARY OSSIFICATION CENTERS IN PROXIMAL END

- For upper end of ulna (olecranon)
  - 9 years (A)
  - 16-17 years (F).

SECONDARY OSSIFICATION CENTERS AT DISTAL END

  - 5 to 6 years (A)
  - 18 years (F).

Anteroposterior (AP) radiograph of left elbow joint shows (Figs 4.2 to 4.4):

- All the epiphyses of lower end of humerus—Fused.
- Epiphysis of head of radius and olecranon—Fused.

Opinion: The age of the individual as per the radiological examination is of adult (more than 16 years).

OTHER IMPORTANT POINTS

- All epiphyses at the proximal and distal ends of long bones unite at about 15 and 16 years of age in females and in 17 and 18 years in males.
- Within the range of two years of age from the appearance and fusion of ossification centers, the age of an individual can be determined.

Anteroposterior (AP) radiograph of left elbow joint shows:

- Conjoint epiphyses of distal end of humerus—not fused.
- Epiphysis of medial and lateral epicondyle—not fused.
- Epiphysis of head of radius—not fused.
- Epiphysis of olecranon—not fused.

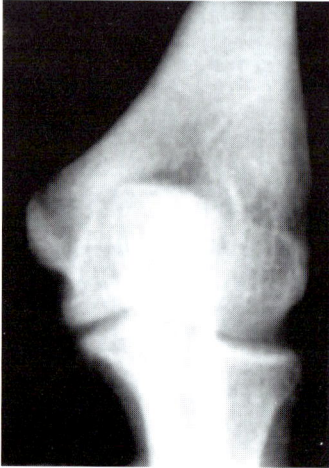

Figure 4.2A: X-ray of left elbow joint—AP view

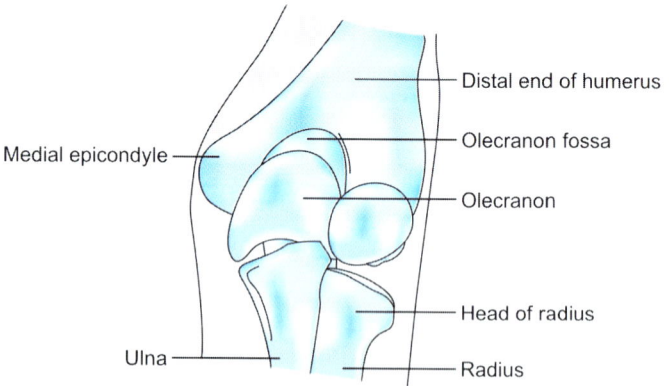

Figure 4.2B: Outline of AP radiograph of left elbow joint

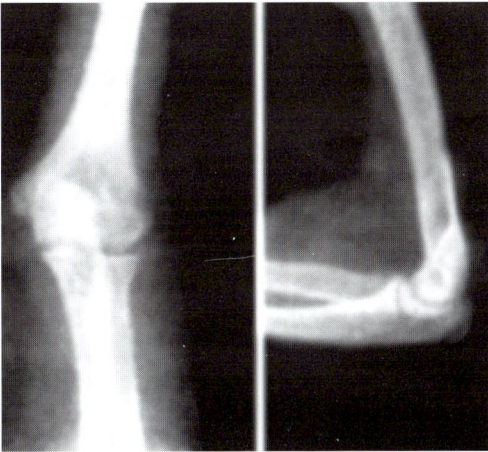

Figure 4.3A: X-ray of left elbow joint—AP and lateral views

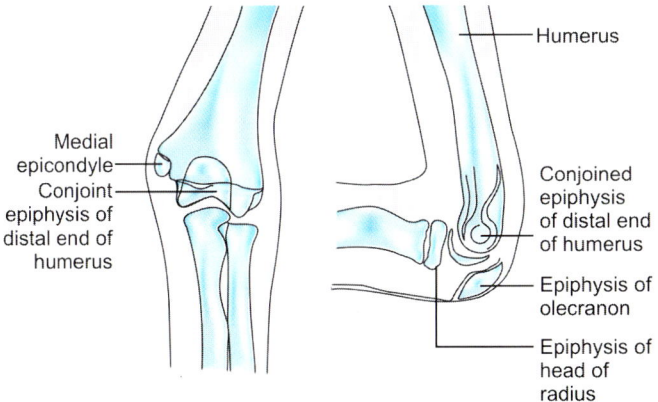

Figure 4.3B: Outline of radiograph of left elbow joint—AP and lateral view

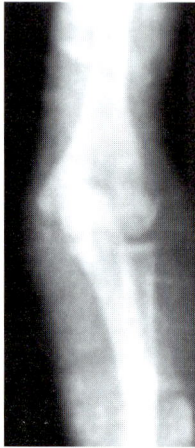

Figure 4.4A: X-ray of left elbow

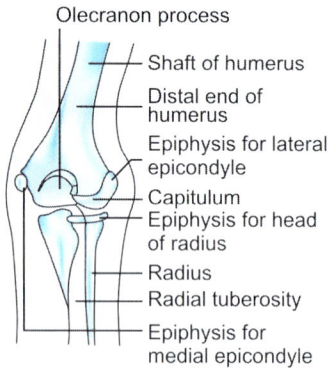

Olecranon process

Shaft of humerus

Distal end of humerus

Epiphysis for lateral epicondyle

Capitulum

Epiphysis for head of radius

Radius

Radial tuberosity

Epiphysis for medial epicondyle

Figure 4.4B: Outline of radiograph left elbow joint—AP view

Opinion: As per the radiological examination of left elbow joint the age of the individual is above 11 years and below 16 years (Lateral epicondyle appeared. Epiphyses of distal end of humerus and proximal ends of radius and ulna are not fused).

Radiograph of left elbow AP and lateral view show:
- Epiphysis of trochlea and capitulum are fused to the shaft of humerus and show recent fusion.
- Medial and lateral epicondyles of lower end of humerus—not fused.
- Epiphysis of head of radius and olecranon—not fused.

Opinion: As per the radiological examination: The age is above 11 years and below 16 years.

Lateral view of left elbow joint radiograph shows (Figs 4.5A and B):
- Epiphyses of lower end of humerus (capitulum, trochlea, medial epicondyle, lateral epicondyle)—not fused.
- Epiphysis of head of radius and olecranon—not fused.

Opinion: As per the radiological examination the age is above 11 years and below 16 years.

Radiograph of right elbow and right wrist AP view show (Figs 4.6A and B):
- Epiphysis of medial epicondyle at lower end of humerus—not fused.
- Epiphysis of base of first metacarpal is completely fused.
- Epiphysis of metacarpal heads are in a stage of recent fusion.

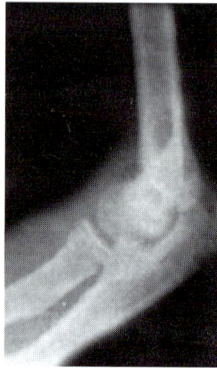

Figure 4.5A: X-ray of left elbow joint—lateral view

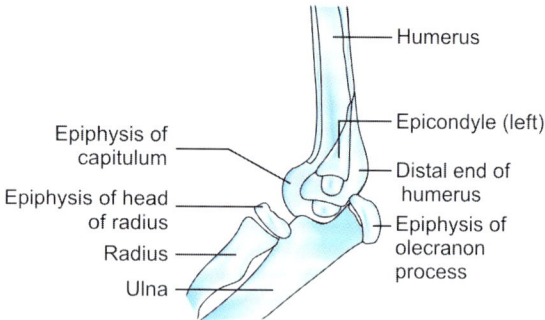

Figure 4.5B: Outline of lateral radiograph of left elbow

- Epiphysis of base of phalanges shows recent fusion and epiphyseal line at the site of fusion.

Opinion: As per the radiological examination: The age is above 16 years and below 18 years.

OTHER IMPORTANT POINT
Sesamoid bone develops in tendon and ligament.

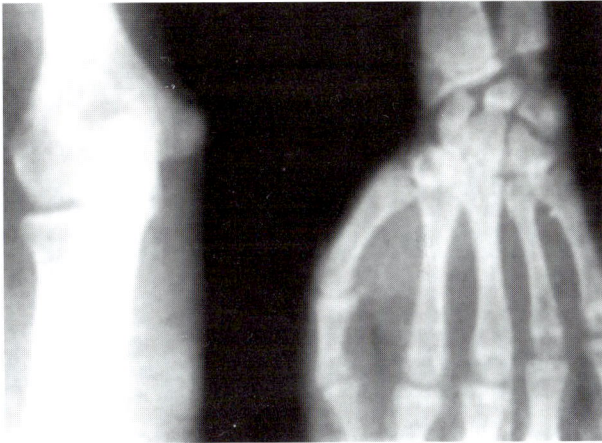

Figure 4.6A: X-ray of right elbow and right wrist

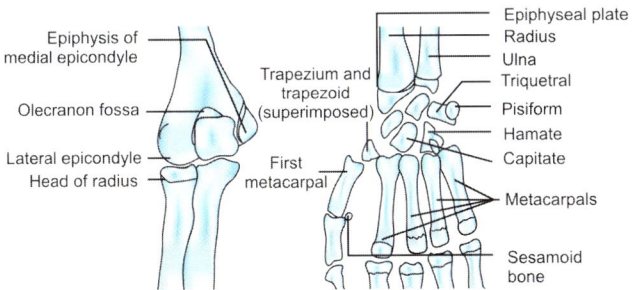

Figure 4.6B: Outline of AP radiograph of right wrist

Anteroposterior radiograph of elbow joint and the wrist joint show (Figs 4.7A and B):

• Epiphysis of distal end of humerus, i.e. capitulum; medial epicondyle; trochlea and lateral epicondyle—not fused.

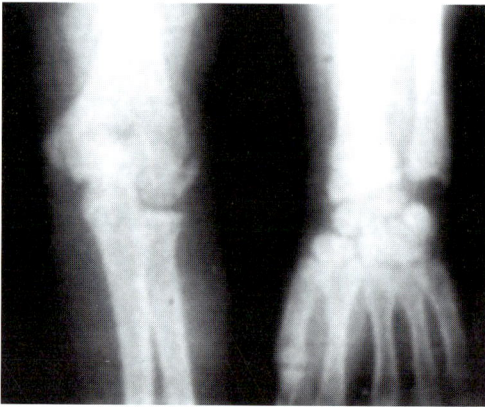

Figure 4.7A: X-ray of left elbow joint and the right wrist joint—AP view

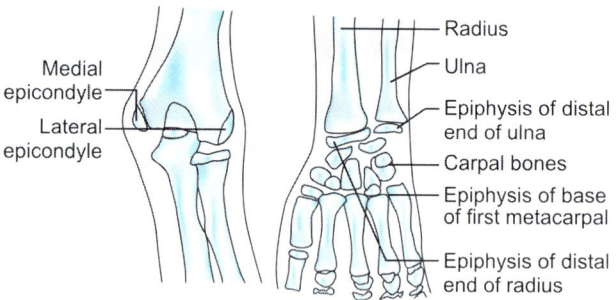

Figure 4.7B: Outline of AP and lateral radiograph of left elbow joint and the right wrist joint

- Epiphysis of head of radius and olecranon of ulna— not fused.
- Epiphysis of distal end of radius and ulna—not fused.
- All eight carpals—ossified.

- Epiphysis of base of first metacarpal bone—not fused.
- Epiphysis of head of other four metacarpal bones—not fused.

Opinion: As per the radiological examination: The age is above 11 years and below 16 years.

Anteroposterior radiograph of left elbow joint shows:

- Conjoint epiphysis of distal end of humerus—not fused.
- Epiphysis of medial epicondyle—not fused.
- Epiphysis for lateral epicondyle—not appeared.
- Epiphysis of head of radius—not fused.
- Epiphysis of olecranon—not appeared.

Opinion: As per the radiological examination: The age is above 5 years and below 9 years.

Anteroposterior and lateral radiographs of left and right elbow joint show (Figs 4.8 and 4.9):

- Epiphysis of capitulum appeared at the distal end of humerus and the other epiphysis at distal end of humerus have not appeared.

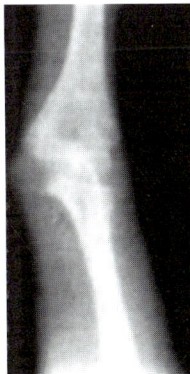

Figure 4.8A: X-ray of left elbow joint—AP view

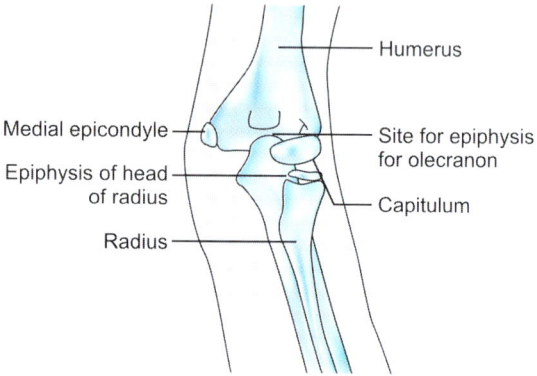

Figure 4.8B: Outline of AP radiograph of right elbow joint

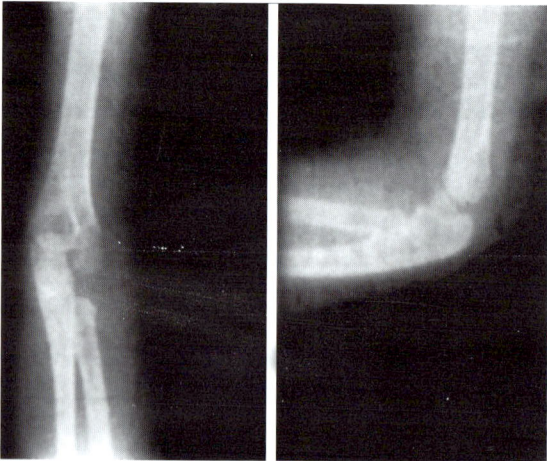

Figure 4.9A: X-ray of left elbow joint—
AP view and right elbow—lateral view

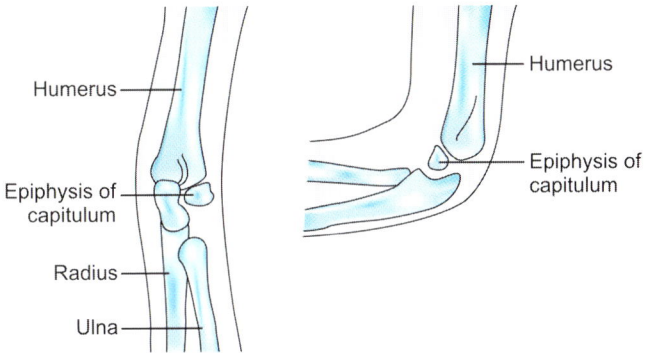

Figure 4.9B: Outline of AP and lateral radiographs of left and right elbow joints

Opinion: As per the radiological examination of elbow joint: The age of the individual is above 1 year and below 5 years.

Chapter 5

Wrist Joint and Hand

■■■■■■■■■■■■■■■■■■■■■■■

DISTAL ENDS OF RADIUS AND ULNA (FIG. 5.1)

Ossification centers: Appearances and fusion.

SECONDARY OSSIFICATION CENTERS

- For lower end of radius : 2 years (A).
  18-19 years (F).
- Lower end of ulna : 5-6 years (A).
  17-18 years (F)

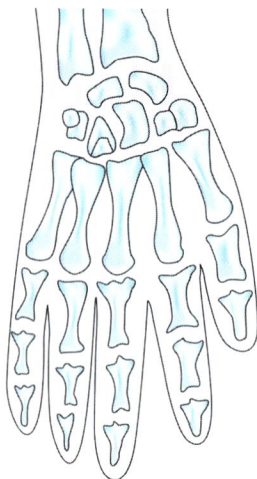

Figure 5.1: Wrist joint and hand

CARPAL BONES

PRIMARY OSSIFICATION CENTERS

None of these are present at birth.
- Capitate : 2 months (A).
- Hamate : 3 months (A).
- Triquetral : 3 years (A).
- Lunate : 4 years (A).
- Trapezium : 4-5 years (A).
- Trapezoid : 4-5 years (A).
- Scaphoid : 4-5 years (A).
- Pisiform : 10-12 years (A).

METACARPAL BONES

PRIMARY CENTER

- First metacarpal bone:
  — Shaft (A) 9 weeks IUL.
- Other four metacarpal bones:
  — Shaft (A) 9 weeks IUL.

SECONDARY CENTER

- Base: 2-3 years (A)
  — 15-17 years (F)
- Head: 1.5-2.5 years (A)
  — 15-19 years (F)

PHALANGES

PRIMARY CENTER

- First phalanges (proximal):
  — Shaft (A) 10 weeks IUL.

- Second phalanges (middle):
  — Shaft (A) 12 weeks IUL.
- Third phalanges (distal):
  — Shaft (A) 8 weeks IUL.

SECONDARY CENTER

Secondary centers in the hand at various ages in both males and females are are shown in Figures 5.2 to 5.13.

- Base: 2 years (A).
  — 15-18 years (F).
- Base: 2-4 years (A)
  — 15-18 years (F).

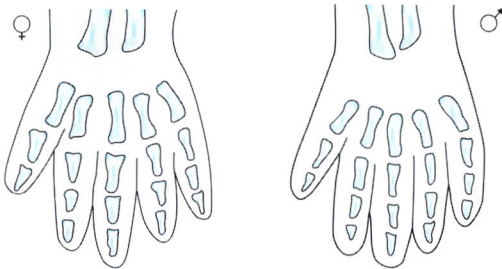

Figure 5.2: Newborn

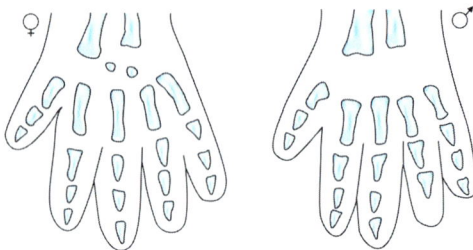

Figure 5.3: Three months

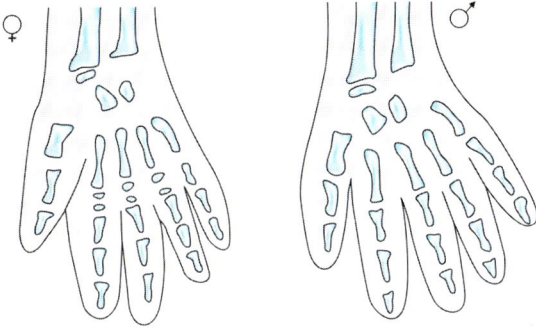

Figure 5.4: One year

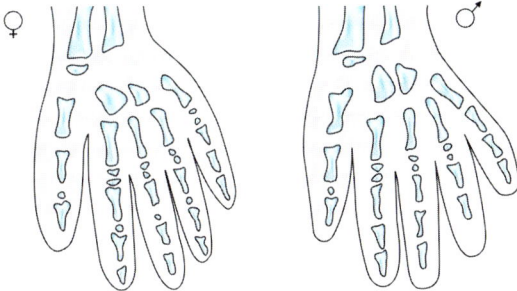

Figure 5.5: Eighteen months

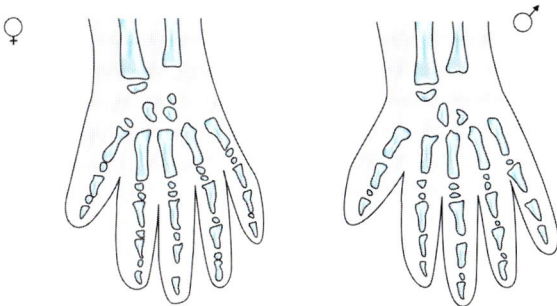

Figure 5.6: Two years

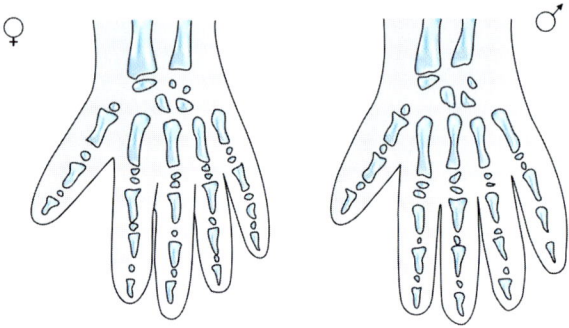

Figure 5.7: Three years

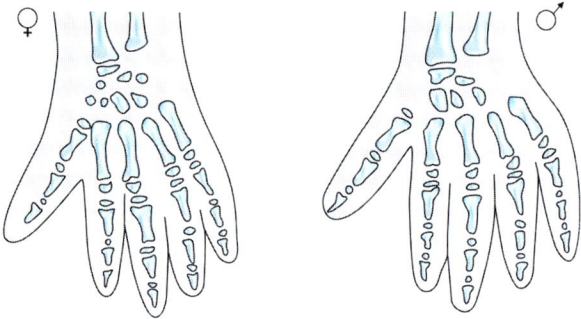

Figure 5.8: Four years

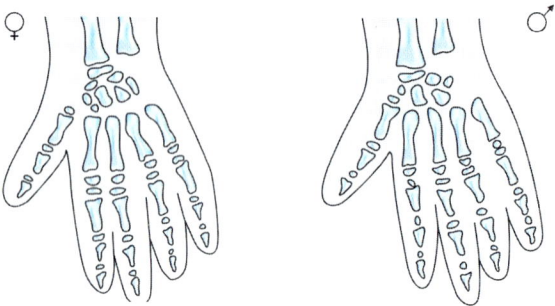

Figure 5.9: Five years

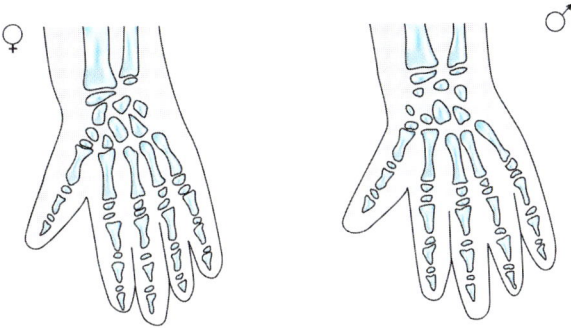

Figure 5.10: Five to six years

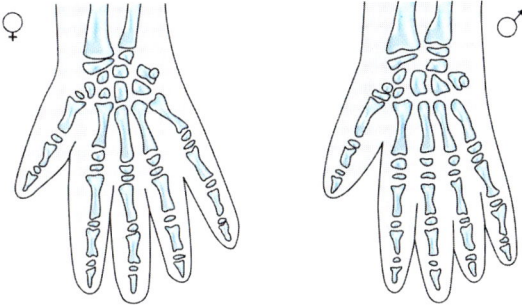

Figure 5.11: 10-12 years

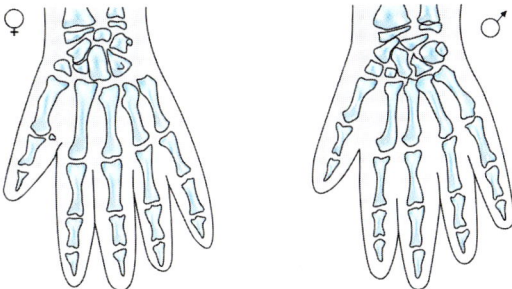

Figure 5.12: 16 and 17 years

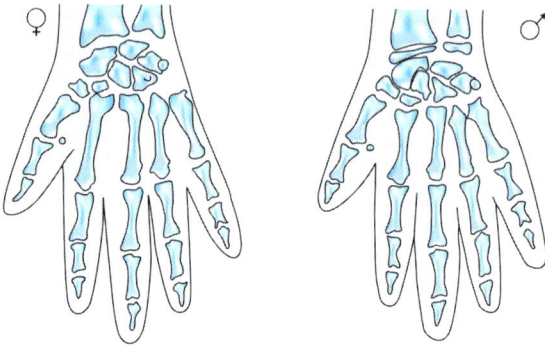

Figure 5.13: 18 and 19 years

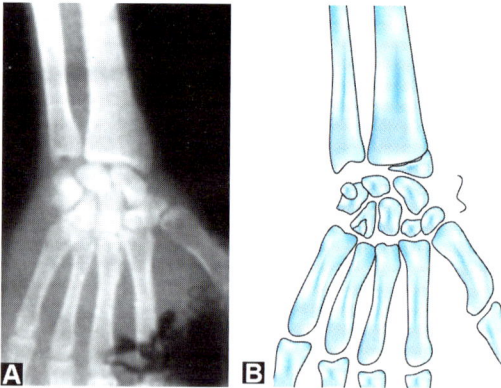

Figures 5.14A and B: (A) X-ray photograph of right wrist—PA view; (B) Outline of PA radiograph of right wrist

Radiograph of right wrist PA view shows: Image of pisiform superimposed on the shadow of triquetral (Figs 5.14 to 5.18).

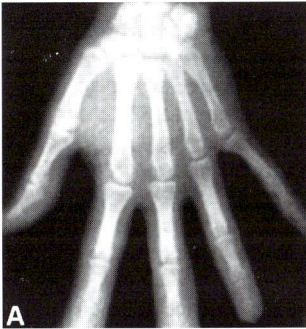

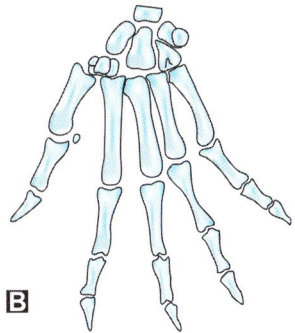

Figures 5.15A and B: (A) X-ray of left wrist and hand—PA view; (B) Outline of PA radiograph of left wrist and hand

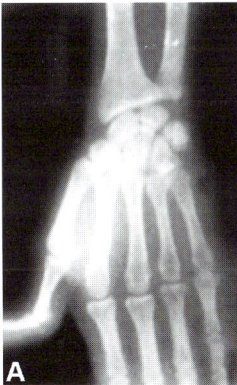

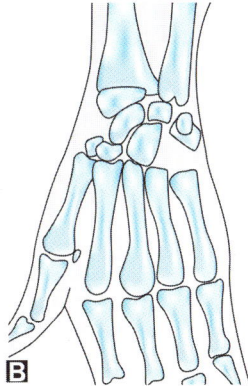

Figures 5.16A and B: (A) X-ray of left wrist—PA view; (B) Outline of PA radiograph of left wrist

Opinion: As per the radiological examination the age of the individual is about 18 years (epiphyseal line is seen in distal end of radius).

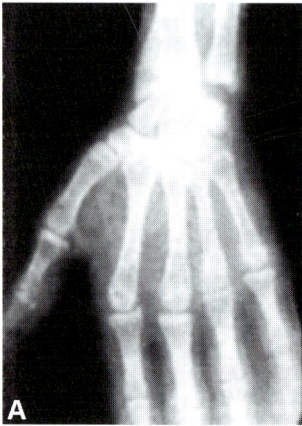

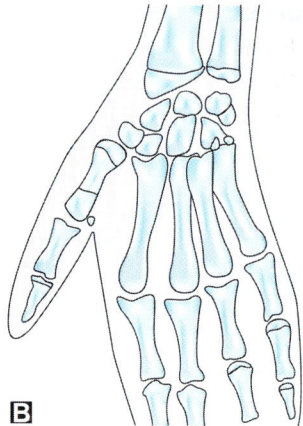

Figures 5.17A and B: (A) X-ray of left wrist joint and hand—PA view; (B) Outline of PA radiograph of left wrist and hand

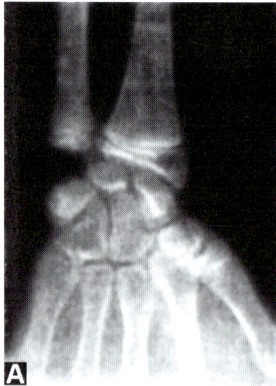

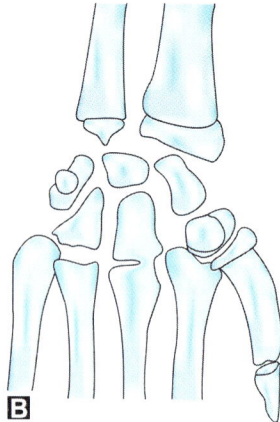

Figures 5.18A and B: (A) X-ray of right wrist—PA view; (B) Outline of PA radiograph of right wrist

Posteroanterior radiograph of right wrist and hand show:
- Eight carpals of wrist joint – ossified.
- Epiphysis of base of first metacarpal and epiphysis of head of other four metacarpals – fused.
- Epiphysis of bases of phalanges – fused.

Opinion: As per the radiological examination: The age of the individual is adult (more than 25 years of age).

OTHER IMPORTANT POINTS

- Eight cartilaginous carpals ossify at different ages.
- The first metacarpophalangeal joints shows one or two sesamoid bones on its anterior side in a radiograph.
- The sesamoid bone is an accessory bone developed from additional ossification center.
- Radiopaque shadows of trapezium and trapezoid overlap each other, partly seen in the X-ray close to the bases of first and second metacarpals of hand.
- The first metacarpophalangeal joint on its anterior side shows one or two sesamoid bones in a radiograph.

Radiograph of left wrist posteroanterior view shows: Image of Pisiform superimposed on the shadow of triquetral.

Opinion: As per the radiological examination:
The age of the individual is between 16 and 18 years.

OTHER IMPORTANT POINTS

- The presence of epiphyseal line at the junction of epiphysis and the diaphysis indicates the age of young adult.

- Proximal row of carpal bones, i.e. scaphoid; lunate; triquetral and pisiform show radiopaque shadows in a skiagram distal to the distal ends of radius and ulna.
- A nearly circular outline shadow of pisiform bone in seen in an X-ray overlying the triquetral.

Posteroanterior radiograph of left wrist and hands shows

- Epiphysis of base of first metacarpal with recent fusion and epiphyseal line.
- Epiphysis of base of each phalange shows recent fusion.

Opinion: As per the radiological examination: The age is above 12 years and below 15 years.

Posteroanterior radiograph of right wrist shows:

- Epiphysis of distal end of radius and ulna—not united. All carpals – ossified.
- Epiphysis of base of first metacarpal—not fused.

Opinion: As per the radiological examination: The age is above 12 years and below 16 years.

OTHER IMPORTANT POINTS

- The image of triquetral is superimposed by pisiform.
- The radiographs are negative images on X-ray films; a dark line at the junction of epiphysis and diaphysis represents epiphyseal cartilaginous plate and the absence of dark line indicates epiphyseal union.

Posteroanterior radiograph of right wrist shows (Fig. 5.19)

- Epiphysis of lower end of radius and ulna: Recent fusion. All carpals ossified.

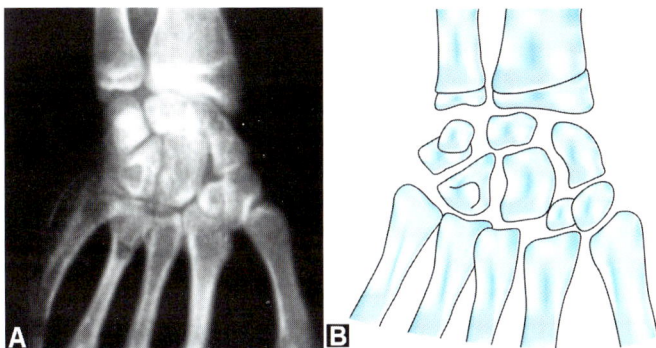

Figures 5.19A and B: (A) X-ray of right wrist—PA view;
(B) Outline of PA radiograph of right wrist

- Epiphysis of base of first metacarpal shows recent
  union with epiphyseal line.

Opinion: As per the radiological examination: The age is
above 15 years and below 17 years.

OTHER IMPORTANT POINTS
• All carpals are cartilaginous at birth. • All the epiphyses of wrist joint are completely fused at 18-20 years of age.

**Posteroanterior radiograph of left wrist and hand shows
(Fig. 5.20)**
- Epiphysis of distal end of radius and ulna: not fused.
- Ossification centers of seven carpals is in advance stage
  of development.
- Ossification center of pisiform has not appeared.
- Epiphysis of base of first metacarpal: not fused.

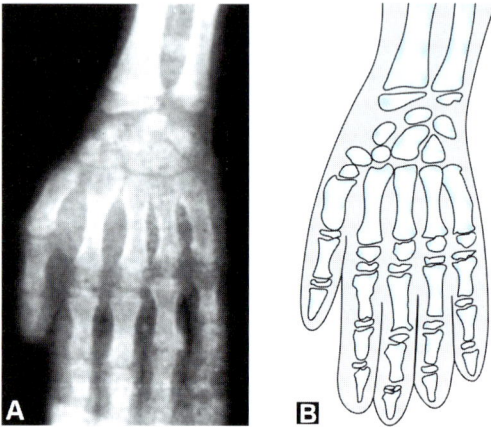

Figures 5.20A and B: (A) X-ray of left wrist and hand—PA view; (B) Outline of PA radiograph of left wrist and hand

- Epiphysis of metacarpal heads: not fused.
- Epiphysis of bases of phalanges: not fused.

Opinion: The age of the individuals is above 5 years and below 11 years as per the radiological examination.

OTHER IMPORTANT POINT
Cartilaginous pisiform does not cast its shadow on the X-ray film below 11 years.

Posteroanterior radiograph of right wrist joint and hand shows (Fig. 5.21)

- Epiphysis of lower end of radius: not fused.
- Epiphysis of lower end of ulna: not appeared.
- Four carpals are in an early stage of development of their ossification centers.

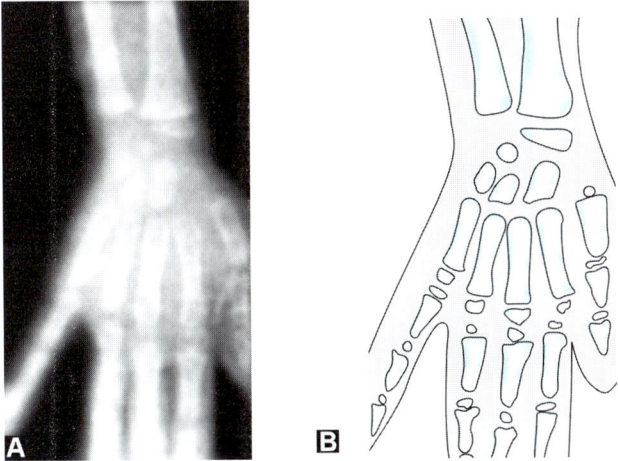

Figures 5.21A and B: X-ray of right wrist joint and hand—PA view; (B) Outline of PA radiograph of right wrist and hand

- Epiphysis of base of first metacarpal is in early stage of development.
- Epiphysis of heads of other four metacarpals are not fused.
- Epiphysis of base of phalanges: not fused.

Opinion: As per the radiological examination of wrist joint and the hand: The age is above 4 years and below 5 years.

OTHER IMPORTANT POINT

Epiphysis is present at the distal end of each four ulnar side metacarpals and for proximal, middle and distal phalanges at their proximal ends.

PA radiograph of right wrist joint and hand shows (Figs 5.22A and B):
- Epiphysis of distal end of radius: Not fused.
- Epiphysis of distal end of ulna: Not appeared.

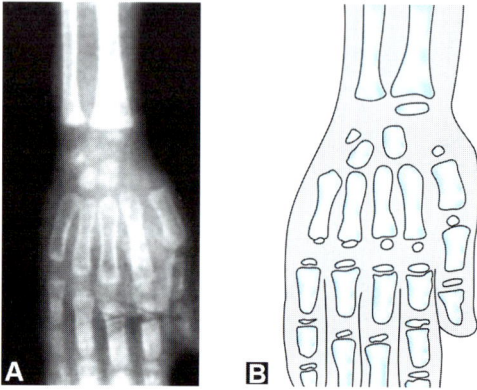

Figures 5.22A and B: (A) X-ray of right wrist joint and hand—PA view; (B) Outline of PA radiograph of right wrist and hand

- Capitate and hamate carpals: Ossified.
- Ossification center of triquetral is in initial stage of development.
- Epiphysis of base of first metacarpal: Not appeared.
- Epiphysis of each metacarpal head and epiphysis of base of each phalange has not fused.

Opinion: Age is about 3 years as per the radiological examination (three cartilaginous carpals are in a stage of ossification).

Radiograph of right wrist joint—lateral view shows (Fig. 5.23):
- Epiphysis of distal end of radius—appeared.
- Cartilaginous carpals, capitate and hamate shows ossification in the earlier stage.
- Epiphysis of distal end of ulna—not appeared.

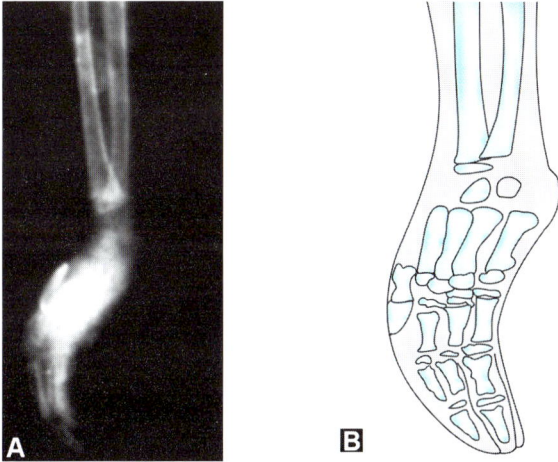

Figures 5.23A and B: (A) X-ray of right wrist joint of a child— lateral view; (B) Outline of lateral radiograph of right wrist joint

Opinion: As per the radiological examination—the age is about 2-3 years and below 5 years.

Chapter 6

Hip Joint and Pelvis

PELVIS/HIP JOINTS (FIG. 6.1)

Ossification centers: Appearance and fusion.

PRIMARY OSSIFICATION CENTER

- Ilium: (A) 8 weeks IUL.
- Pubis: (A) 18 weeks IUL.
- Ischium: (A) 12 weeks IUL.

SECONDARY OSSIFICATION CENTER

- Ilium: Iliac crest:
  - 14 years (A).
  - 19-20 years (F).

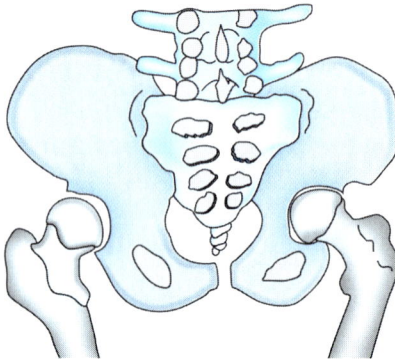

Figure 6.1: Pelvis/hip joints
(Ossification centers: Appearance and fusion)

- Triradiate cartilage (Y-shaped)
  - 13 years (A).
  - 15 years (F).
- Pubis puberty (A).
  - 20 years (F).
- Ischium:
  - 16 Years (A).
  - 20-21 years (F).

PROXIMAL END OF FEMUR (SECONDARY CENTER)

- Head of femur   :   1 year (A).
                          :   17-18 years (F).
- Greater trochanter   :   4 years (A).
                          :   17-18 years (F).
- Lesser trochanter   :   12-14 years (A).
                          :   17-18 years (F).

Anteroposterior radiograph of male pelvis shows (Figs 6.2A and B):
- Epiphysis of iliac crest—fused.
- Y-shaped cartilage in the acetabulum—ossified and fused.

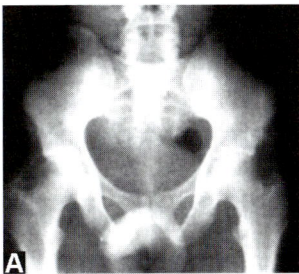

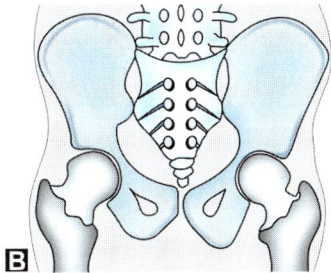

Figures 6.2A and B: (A) X-ray of male pelvis—AP view; (B) Outline of AP radiograph of male pelvis

- Inferior ramus of the pubis and ischial ramus are fused with bony union.
- Epiphyses of proximal end of femur, i.e. head; greater trochanter and lesser trochanter are fused to the shaft.
- All the segments of sacrum are united.
- Articulation of coccyx with the sacrum is seen at the sacral apex.

Opinion: As per the radiological examination: The age of male adult is above 21 years and below 25 years.

Anteroposterior radiograph of female pelvis shows (Figs 6.3A and B):
- Epiphysis of iliac crest in a stage of fusion.
- Y-shaped cartilage in the acetabulum—ossified and fused.
- Epiphyses of proximal end of femur are fused.

Opinion: As per the radiological examination: The age of female adult is above 20 years and below 25 years.

OTHER IMPORTANT POINT
The fusion of epiphyses in bones takes place two years earlier in the female than in the male.

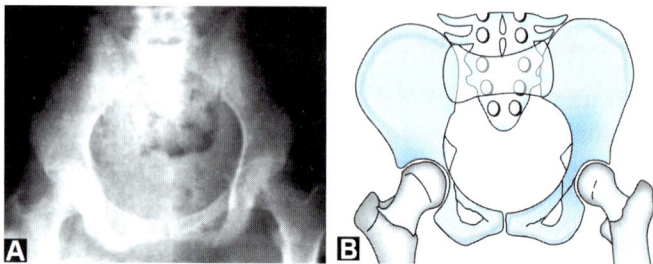

Figures 6.3A and B: (A) X-ray of female pelvis—AP view; (B) Outline of AP radiograph of female pelvis

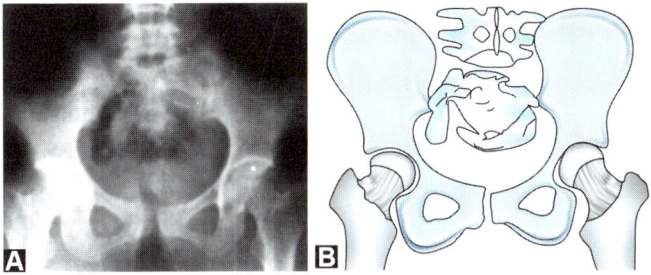

Figures 6.4A and B: (A) X-ray of female pelvis—AP view;
(B) Outline of AP radiograph of female pelvis

Anteroposterior radiograph of female pelvis shows (Figs 6.4A and B):

- Epiphysis of iliac crest of ilium—fused completely. Triradiate cartilage in the acetabulum. Y-shaped cartilage—ossified and united the ilium, ischium and the pubis.
- Epiphysis of ischial tuberosity—appeared but not fused.
- Inferior ramus of the pubis is united with the ischial ramus with the bony union.
- Epiphysis of the proximal end of femur, i.e. head; greater trochanter and lesser tronchanter are fused to the shaft.
- Neck of femur shows extension of cone of lamellar pattern of spongy bone to the anatomical neck.

Opinion: As per the radiological examination: The age of female adult is about 20 years (above 16 years and below 21 years).

Anteroposterior radiograph of left hip joint shows (Figs 6.5A and B):

- Lamellar pattern of cancellous bone in the neck of femur.

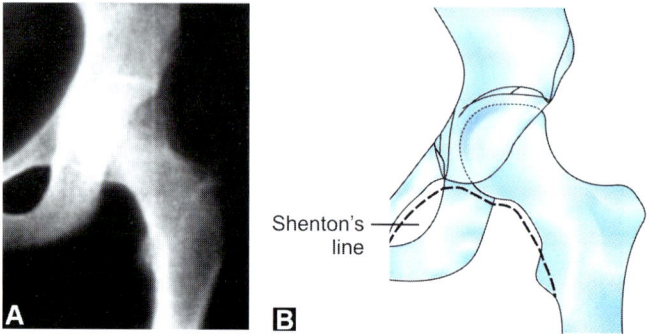

Figures 6.5A and B: (A) X-ray of left hip joint—AP view; (B) Outline of AP radiograph of left hip joint

- The cone of medullary cavity from the shaft is extending into the neck more than its middle third.

Opinion: As per the radiological examination: The age is about 18 years (17-18 years: Lesser trochanter shows "partial union".

OTHER IMPORTANT POINTS

- Architecture of bony trabeculae of spongy bone in the neck of femur with the cone of medullary cavity can be visualized in the X-ray film.
- Intertrochanteric crest and lines are seen superimposed in an X-ray.

Anteroposterior radiograph of right hip joint and pelvic bone shows (Figs 6.6A and B):
- Epiphyses of iliac crest—not fused.
- Triradiated cartilage in the acetabulum—not ossified completely.

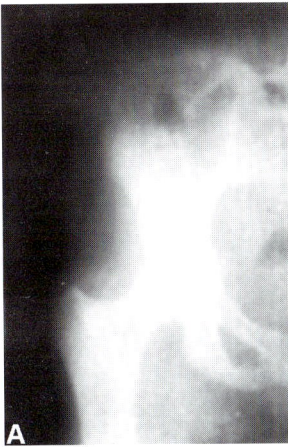

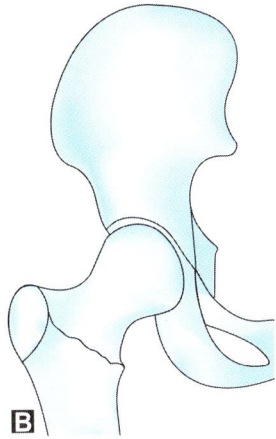

Figures 6.6A and B: (A) X-ray of right hip joint and pelvic bone—AP view; (B) Outline of AP radiograph of right hip joint and pelvic bone

- Ischial ramus is fused with the inferior ramus of pubis.
- Epiphysis of greater trochanter of femur—recently fused.

Opinion: As per the radiological examination: The age is about 18 years (above 18 years and below 20 years).

OTHER IMPORTANT POINT

The site of union of inferior ramus of pubis with ischial ramus is marked by localized thickening.

Radiograph of pelvis—AP view shows (Figs 6.7A and B):
- Epiphysis of iliac crest—not appeared.
- Triradiate cartilage in acetabulum—not ossified and not united the ischium, pubis and ilium.

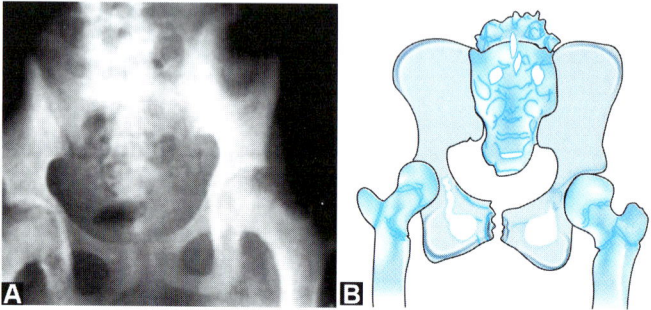

Figures 6.7A and B: (A) X-ray of pelvis—AP view; (B) Outline of AP radiograph of pelvis

- Inferior ramus of pubis is fused with ischial ramus as the binding cartilage is ossified.
- Epiphysis of head of femur, greater trochanter and lesser trochanter—not fused.
- Lesser trochanter is in beginning stage of ossification.

Opinion: The age is above 12 years and below 14 years (sacral vertebrae are also not fused. They fuse from 21-25 years completely).

OTHER IMPORTANT POINTS

- Sacrum is formed by fusion of five sacral vertebrae. Line of fusion shows raised transverse ridge.
- Symphyseal surface having horizontal bony ridges grooves and irregular surface (billowing) can be visualized in radiographs, which indicate age.

Anteroposterior radiograph of pelvis and hip joint show (Figs 6.8A and B):
- Epiphysis of crest of ilium—not appeared.
- Triradiate cartilage in acetabulum—not ossified.

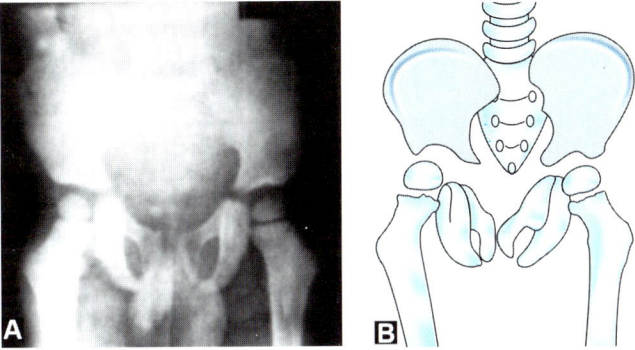

Figures 6.8A and B: (A) X-ray of pelvis and hip joint—AP view; (B) Outline of AP radiograph of pelvis and hip joint

- Inferior ramus of the pubis—not united with the ischial ramus by bony union.
- Epiphysis of head of femur appeared; greater trochanter and lesser trochanter—not appeared.

Opinion: As per the radiological examination: The age is about 2 years (above 1 year and below 4 years—greater trochanter not appear).

Chapter 7

Knee Joint

■ ■

Ossification centers: Appearance (A) and fusion (F).

DISTAL END OF FEMUR (FIG. 7.1)

PRIMARY CENTER

- In shaft of femur appears in 8 weeks IUL.
- Proximal end of tibia   :   At birth (A)
                                        :   18-19 years (F).
- Proximal end of fibula   :   At 4 years (A)
                                        :   18-19 years (F).

SECONDARY CENTER

- Ninth month (A).
- 18-19 years (F).

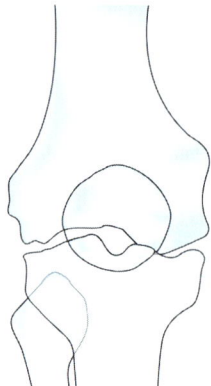

Figure 7.1: Knee joint

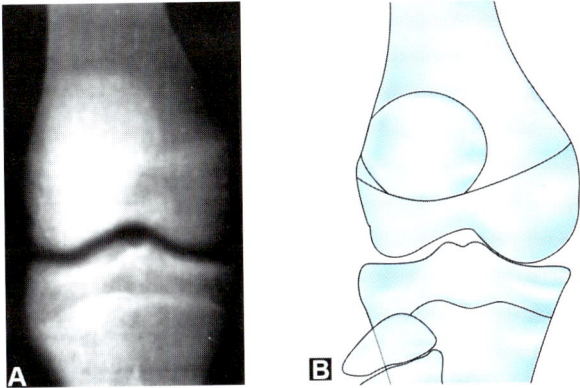

Figures 7.2A and B: (A) X-ray of right knee joint—AP view;
(B) Outline of AP radiograph of right knee

Anteroposterior radiograph of right knee joint shows (Figs 7.2A and B):

- Epiphysis of lower end of femur—not fused.
- Epiphysis of upper end of tibia and fibula—not fused.

Opinion: The age is above 4 years and below 18 years.

OTHER IMPORTANT POINTS

- The shadow of patella is superimposed on distal end of femur.
- Patella is the largest sesamoid bone in the body.
- Cartilaginous growth plate is interposed between the diaphysis and the epiphysis.
- The medial and lateral menisci are semilunar cartilages covering the articular surfaces of proximal end of tibia in the knee joint. Lateral meniscus is nearly circular and smaller than the medial meniscus, which is oval and larger.

- Ossification in the patella begins at the age of three years.
- The presence of ossification center in lower end of femur in an abandoned baby establishes that the child was viable at birth; as the center appears before birth.
- Bone increases in length at growth plate and reach its maturity.

Anteroposterior radiograph of right knee—AP view shows (Fig. 7.3):

- Epiphysis of lower end of femur and upper end of tibia—not fused.
- Epiphysis of proximal end of fibula—not appeared.
- Epiphysis of patella—not appeared.

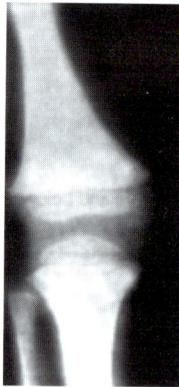

Figure 7.3: X-ray of right knee—AP view

Opinion: As per the radiological examination: The age is above 1 year and below 3 years.

OTHER IMPORTANT POINT

Absence of shadow of patella indicates the presence of cartilaginous patella, which ossifies at the age of 3 years.

Chapter 8

Ankle Joint and Foot

ANKLE JOINT (FIGS 8.1A AND B)

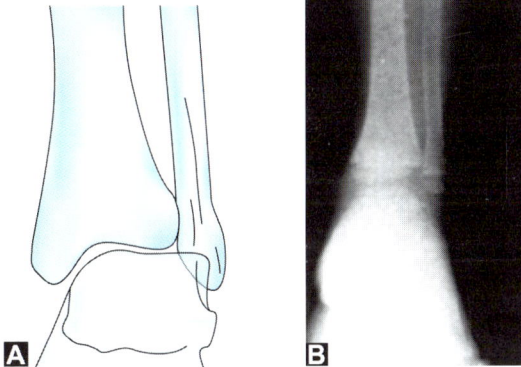

Figures 8.1A and B: (A) Ankle joint ossification centers: (appearance and fusion) (B) X-ray of right ankle joint—AP view

SECONDARY CENTER

- Lower end of tibia
  - One year (A)
  - 16-17 years (F)
- Lower end of fibula
  - One year (A)
  - 16-17 years (F)

- Talus (primary center)
  - — Seventh month (A) IUL.

AP radiograph of right ankle joint shows: Epiphysis of lower end of tibia and lower end of fibula: appeared and not fused.

Opinion: As per the radiological examination: The age is about 1 year.

FOOT BONES (FIGS 8.2A TO C)

TARSAL BONES

Primary Centers

- Calcaneum: Fifth month IUL (A)
- Talus: Seventh month IUL (A)
- Cuboid: Ninth month (A) at birth
- Navicular: 3 years (A)
- Medial cuneiform: 2 years (A).

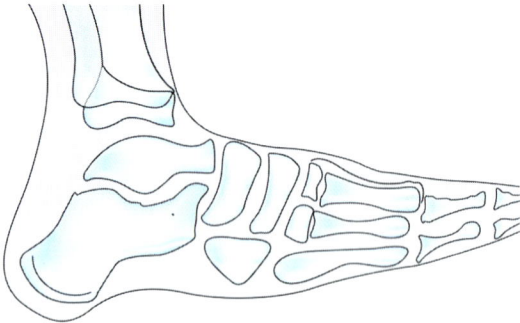

Figure 8.2A: Bones of right foot and ankle (distal ends of tibia and fibula, calcaneum, talus, navicular, cuneiforms, metatarsals and phalanges)

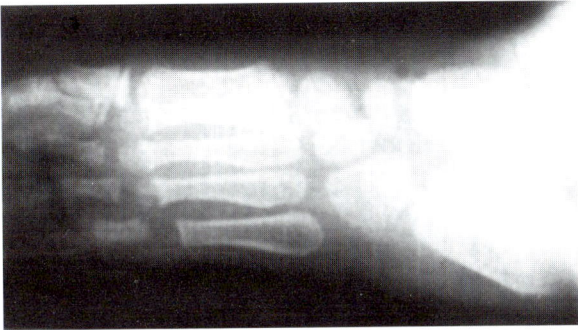

Figure 8.2B: Primary and secondary ossification centers of right foot bones

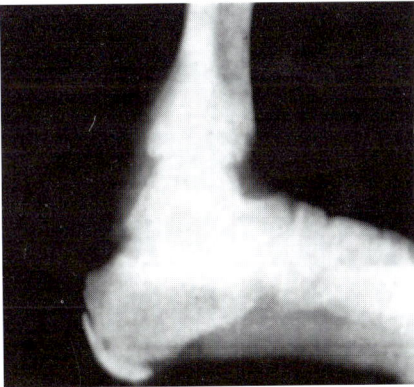

Figure 8.2C: Ossification of secondary center for epiphysis of posterior part of calcaneum

- Middle cuneiform: 3 years (A).
- Lateral cuneiform: 1 year (A).

Secondary Centers

- Epiphysis of posterior surface of calcaneum:
  - 6-8 years (A)
  - 14-16 years (F).

METATARSAL BONES

Primary Centers

- First metatarsal bone
  Shaft: 10 weeks IUL.
- Second to fifth.
  Shafts: 9 weeks IUL.

Secondary Centers

- Base: 3 years (A).
  17-20 years (F).
- Heads: 3-4 years (A).
  17-20 years (F).

PHALANGES

Primary Centers

- Proximal phalanges:
  Shafts: 11-15 weeks (A)
- Middle phalanges:
  Shafts: 13 weeks (A)
- Distal phalanges:
  Shafts: 9-12 weeks (A)

Secondary Centers

- Bases: 2-8 years (A)
  18 years (F)
- Bases: 3-6 years (A)
  18 years (F)
- Bases: 6 years (A)
  18 years (F)

Chapter 9

Skull Vault and Suture Closure

■ ■

VAULT OF THE SKULL AND CLOSURE OF THE SUTURES

Anteroposterior radiograph of skull shows (Figs 9.1A and B)

- Metopic suture (interfrontal) – not closed.
- Sockets of incisor teeth in upper jaw are empty and suggests postmortem shedding.

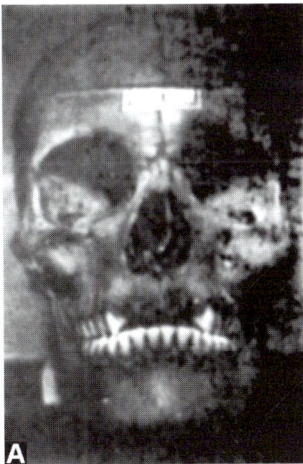

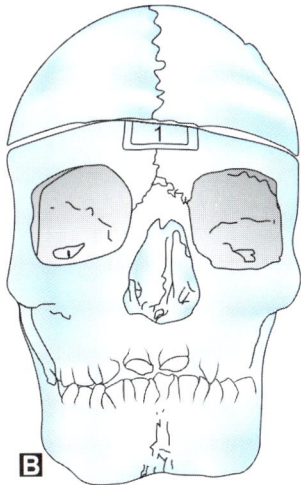

Figures 9.1A and B: (A) X-ray of skull—AP view; (B) Outline of AP radiograph of skull

- The circular cut in the vault indicates first postmortem examination.
- Scale on the forehead indicates super imposition photography done for identity.
- Adult skull with persistent metopic suture.

OTHER IMPORTANT POINTS

- At birth two frontal bones are separated by metopic suture. In 90% it is obliterated by 6-8 years of life.
- Every skull varies in its shape.
- In an individual having a persistent metopic suture; both frontal sinus are usually absent.

Lateral radiograph of skull shows (Figs 9.2A and B):

- Sutures of vault: Not closed (endocranially and ectocranially).

Opinion: The age is about 20-22 years.

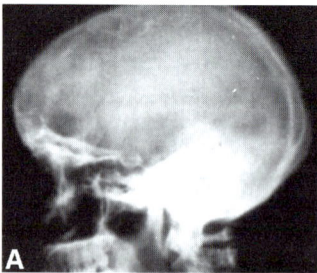

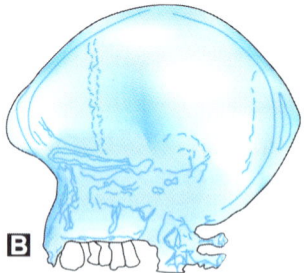

Figures 9.2A and B: (A) X-ray of skull—lateral view; (B) Outline of skull—lateral view

OTHER IMPORTANT POINTS

- Crista galli is the crest bony elevation in the median plane of cribriform plate of ethmoid bone.
- Interlocking of serrated margins in lambdoid suture indicate nonclosure both endocranially as well as ectocranially.
- Skull vault sutures closed early on their inner table than on the outer side.
- Anterior one-third of sagittal suture closes at about 40-50 years and posterior one-third at about 30-40 years.
- Upper half of coronal suture closes at about 50-60 years and lower half at about 40-60 years.

Chapter 10

Mixed Dentition

■ ■

Lateral radiograph of skull and lower jaw of a child shows (Figs 10.1A and B): Mixed dentition permanent first molar tooth is formed behind the temporary second molar tooth. The permanent incisors are also in early stages of development below the temporary incisors in lower and upper jaws.

Opinion: The age is about 6-7 years (child).

OTHER IMPORTANT POINT
Anterior fontanelle close at one and half years.

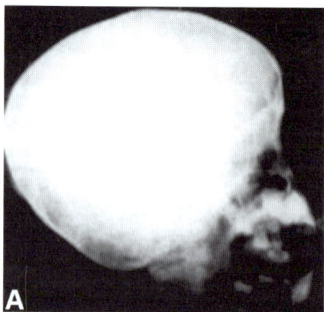

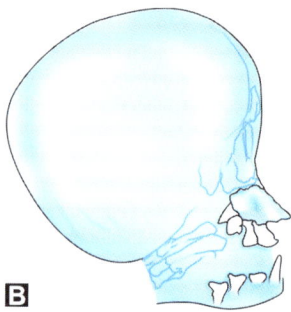

Figures 10.1A and B: (A) X-ray of skull and lower jaw of a child—lateral view; (B) Outline of skull and lower jaw of a child—lateral view

Chapter 11

Collar Bone

Radiograph of left collar bone (inner end) PA view shows: Epiphysis of sternal end of clavicle has appeared and well developed. It is not fused completely (Figs 11.1A and B).

Opinion: As per the radiological examination, the age is about 21 years (epiphyseal line of fusion is visible).

OTHER IMPORTANT POINTS

- Clavicle is the first bone in body to undergo ossification, which is intramembranous.
- Epiphysis is present at the sternal end of collar bone only.

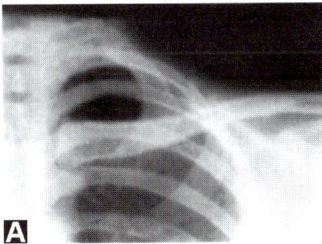

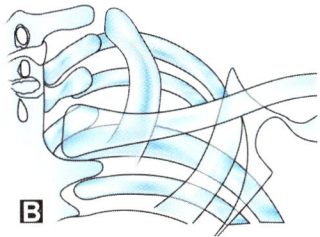

Figures 11.1A and B: (A) X-ray of left collar bone (sternal end)—PA view; (B) Outline of left collar bone (sternal end)—PA view

Chapter 12

Hyoid Bone

■ ■

X-rays (lateral view) hyoid bone and cervical vertebrae; hyoid bone and laryngeal cartilages and hyoid bone, larynx, trachea and cervical vertebrae are shown in Figures 12.1 and 12.2.

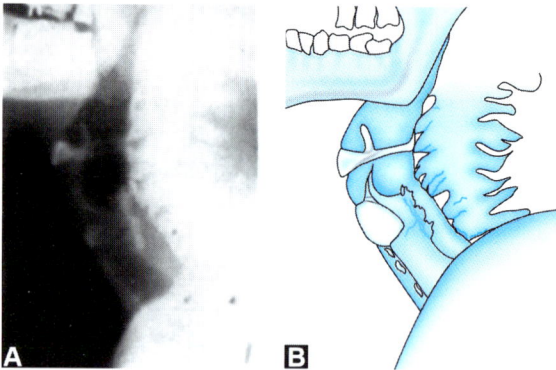

Figures 12.1A and B: (A) X-ray of hyoid bone and cervical vertebrae; (B) Outline of hyoid bone and laryngeal cartilages showing calcification—lateral view

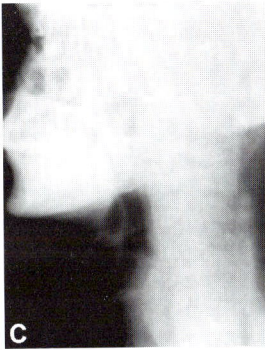

Figure 12.1C: X-ray of hyoid bone and laryngeal cartilages showing calcification—lateral view

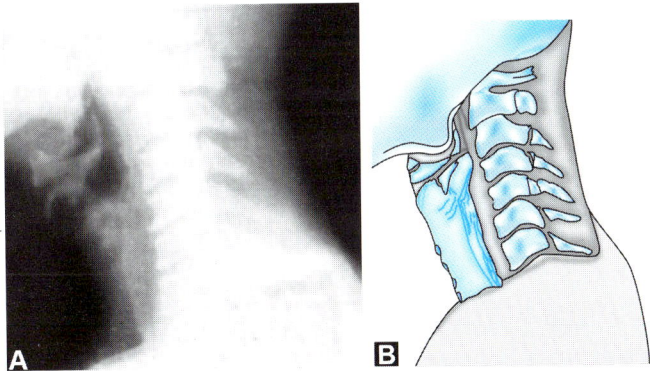

Figures 12.2A and B: (A) X-ray of hyoid bone, larynx, trachea and cervical vertebrae—lateral view; (B) Outline of lateral radiograph of hyoid bone, larynx, trachea and cervical vertebrae—lateral view

OTHER IMPORTANT POINTS

- First CV consists of anterior and posterior arch and two lateral masses. The anterior arch has an anterior tubercle.
- Second CV has odontoid process and spinous process, which is bifid.
- The superior surface of body of each cervical vertebra is saddle shaped and the inferior surface concave. A projection from its anterior margin overlaps the anterior surface of intervertebral disk.
- Larynx in an adult lies opposite the third to sixth cervical vertebrae.
- Ossification of laryngeal cartilages occurs at 45-50 years.

Lateral radiograph of hyoid bone and cervical vertebrae of neck shows: Body and greater cornuae are not fused; soft tissue shadow of larynx vestibular fold above the sinus of larynx and vocal folds below enclosing the space of glottis (Figs 12.3 and 12.4).

Opinion: Age below 35-40 years.

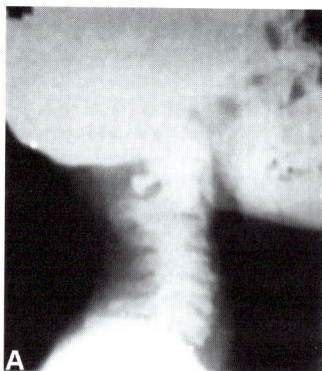

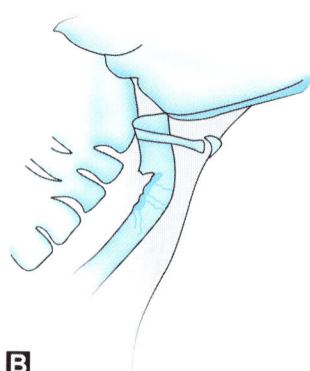

Figures 12.3A and B: (A) X-ray of hyoid bone and cervical vertebrae of neck—lateral view; (B) Outline of lateral radiograph of hyoid bone and cervical vertebrae of neck

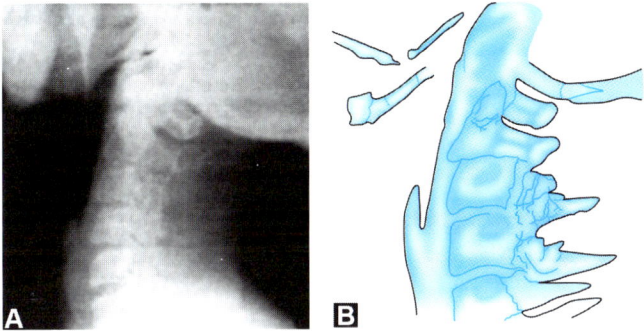

Figures 12.4A and B: (A) X-ray of hyoid bone and cervical vertebrae of neck—lateral view. Lateral radiograph of hyoid bone and cervical vertebrae; (B) Outline of lateral radiograph of hyoid bone and cervical vertebrae of neck

OTHER IMPORTANT POINTS

- First CV consists of anterior and posterior arch and two lateral masses. The anterior arch has an anterior tubercle.
- Second CV has odontoid process and spinous process, which is bifid.
- The superior surface of body of each cervical vertebra is saddle shaped and the inferior surface concave. A projection from its anterior margin overlaps the anterior surface of intervertebra disk.
- Larynx in an adult lies opposite the 3-6th cervical vertebrae.
- Ossification of laryngeal cartilages occurs at 45-50 years.

Lateral radiograph of lower jaw and the neck shows (Figs 12.5A and B)

- Body of hyoid bone not united with greater cornua.
- Soft tissue shadow of larynx with the epiglottis is also seen anterior to the cervical vertebrae.

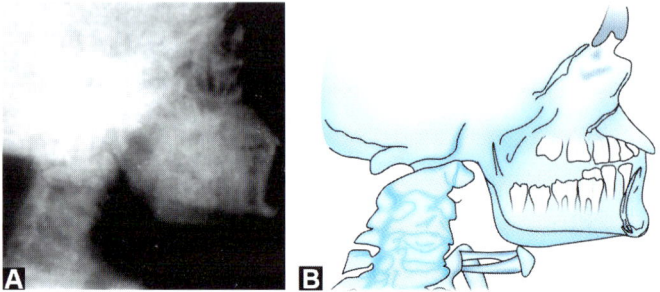

Figures 12.5A and B: (A) X-ray of lower jaw and neck—lateral view; (B) Outline of lateral radiograph of lower jaw and the neck

- The epiglottis is seen projecting above the hyoid bone.

Opinion: Age below 30-35 years.

OTHER IMPORTANT POINTS

- Body of hyoid bone lies at the level of body of fourth CV and greater cornuae extended from the body postero-superiorly.
- Greater cornuae are obliquely situated.
- Epiglottis is a leaf-like elastic fibrocartilage having pitted surface and projects above the level of hyoid bone. It acts as a lid over the larynx while swallowing bolus of food.
- Vocal cords are situated in the middle of larynx.

Lateral radiograph of hyoid bone and cervical vertebrae shows (Figs 12.6A and B): Ossified joints on either side of body of hyoid bone; soft tissue shadow of thyroid

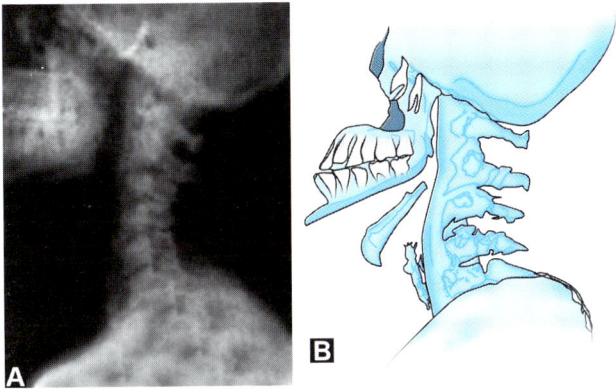

Figures 12.6A and B: (A) X-ray of hyoid bone and cervical vertebrae—lateral view; (B) Outline of lateral radiograph of hyoid bone and cervical vertebrae

cartilage; cricoid cartilage and tracheal rings, which are in a stage of ossification.

Opinion: Age about 35-40 years.

OTHER IMPORTANT POINTS

- Intervertebral disk composed of concentric rings of fibro-cartilage and central pulp (nucleus pulposus).
- All cervical vertebrae (except the seventh) transmit vertebral artery through foramen transversarium, venous plexus and sympathetic plexus. The foramen transversarium of seventh cervical vertebra transmits only venous plexus.

Chapter 13

Sternum

Lateral radiograph of sternum shows: All the four body segments of sternum: Fused. Manubrium sterni is not united with the body of sternum. Xiphisternum is not united to the body of sternum (Figs 13.1A and B).

Opinion: Age above 25 years and below 40 years (sternal segments are fused; xiphisternum is not fused to the body of sternum).

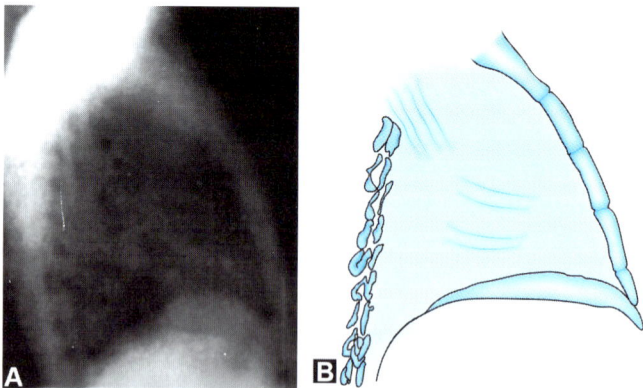

Figures 13.1A and B: (A) X-ray of sternum—lateral view; (B) Outline of lateral radiograph of sternum

OTHER IMPORTANT POINTS

- The sternum consists of outer compact layer of bone and inner spongy substance.
- Four middle pieces of sternum fuse with one another from below up wards from 14 to 25 years of age. The site of fusion is marked by a transverse bony ridge on inner side of the sternum between the sternal segments.
- Manubrium sterni unites with the body in old age (about 50 years).
- Xiphoid process of sternum unites with the body of sternum at about 40 years.
- Manubrium sterni lies at the level of bodies of t3, t4 vertebrae and the body of sternum at the level of t5 to t9 vertebrae.
- The posterior surface of manubrium sterni in its lower part is in relation to arch of aorta.
- Xiphoid process may be pointed, bifid; perforated; curved or deflected to one side.

2

Traumatic Bone Fracture and Dislocation Injuries in Medicolegal Cases

Chapter 14

Traumatic Bone Fracture and Dislocation Injuries in Medicolegal Cases

■ ■

Radiograph of skull, facial bones and frontal view for frontal sinus are shown in Figures 14.1 and 14.2, and radiograph shown posteroanterior view (Fig 14.3) of chest and upper abdomen.

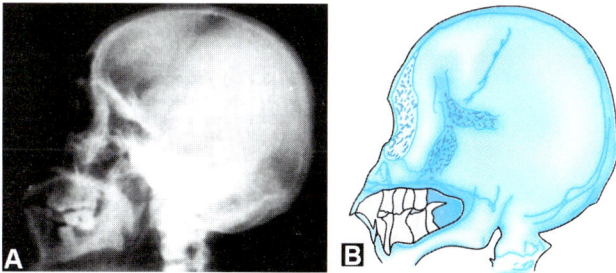

Figures 14.1A and B: (A) Lateral radiograph of skull and facial bones; (B) Outline of lateral radiograph of skull and facial bones

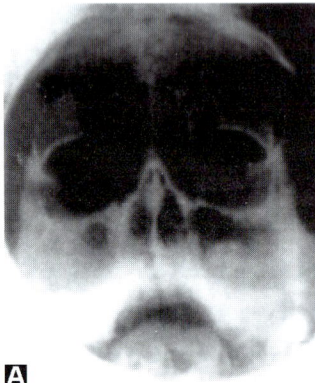
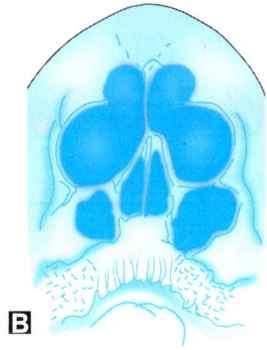

Figures 14.2A and B: (A) Radiograph of skull: Frontal view for frontal sinuses; (B) Outline of radiograph of skull showing frontal sinuses

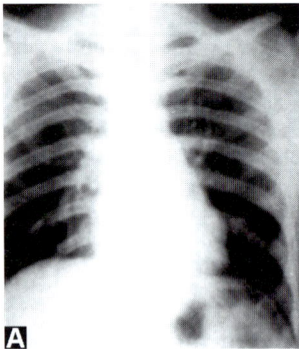
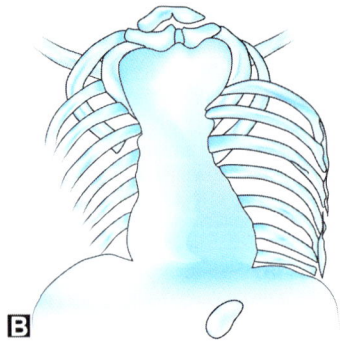

Figures 14.3A and B: (A) Posteroanterior view of radiograph of chest and upper abdomen; (B) Outline of posteroanterior view of radiograph of chest and upper abdomen

INJURIES OF THE FACIAL SKELETON

FRACTURE OF THE NASAL BONES

Nasal bones are commonly fractured from fist blows in criminal assaults and reveal local deformity.

FRACTURES OF THE MAXILLARY BONES

The maxillae are fractured in forcible falls from height and in vehicular road accidents.

FRACTURES OF THE MANDIBLE

In criminal assaults and in accidental falls the mandible is fractured at its weakest point in its body at the deep canine socket on either side from localized impacts of blunt force.

The lower jaw may be fractured at the junction of the ramus with the body in blunt force injuries. Fracture at the symphysis menti is caused mostly in railway and road accidents. Fracture of the neck of mandible is caused by the blunt force injury with local deformity but is rare (Fig. 14.3C).

INJURIES TO THE FRONT OF THE NECK

HYOID BONE FRACTURES

An ossified hyoid bone in an elderly individual may be fractured at the junction of the body and greater cornua. The hyoid bone fractures also occurs as:
a. Inward compression fractures,
b. Anteroposterior compression fractures and
c. Avulsion fractures.

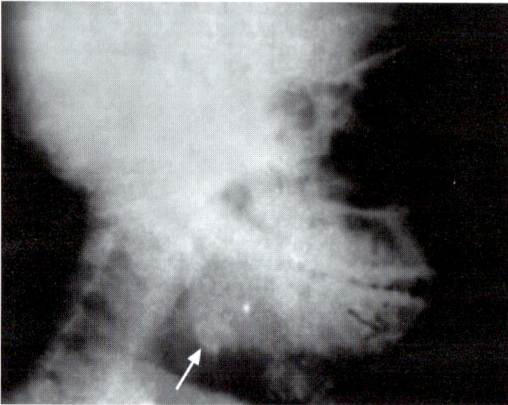

Figure 14.3C: Splintered metal fragments. Blast injury mandible (open reduction with dental wiring)

Inward Compression Fractures

The inward compression fracture is common in throttling in an elderly individual. The hyoid bone is fractured in its greater cornu at the junction of its medial two-third and the lateral one-third. The posterior fragments of the greater cornuae are displaced and show convergence inwards and the periosteum is torn on the outside at the fracture sites. Antemortem fracture reveal bleeding at the fracture site and below the periosteum. A fracture at the joint between greater cornu and the body of hyoid bone also may occur in the elderly individual above 45 years of age due to calcification at the joints. The fracture may be unilateral or bilateral.

Anteroposterior Compression Fracture

The anteroposterior compression fracture is common in strangulation. The greater cornua is fractured at the junction of medial two-third and lateral one-third with outward displacement of the posterior fragments of the greater cornua. The greater cornuae show divergence and tearing of periosteum on innersides at the fracture sites. The fracture may be unilateral or bilateral.

Avulsion Fracture

Avulsion fracture is a traction fracture occurring due to muscular pull on the hyoid bone in hanging. The hyoid bone is forced backwards against the cervical vertebrae and gets fractured in its greater horns.

LARYNGEAL SKELETON FRACTURES

Mainly the thyroid cartilage and the cricoid cartilage are broken. The superior horns of the thyroid cartilage are commonly fractured in throttling and strangulation. In a blunt force injury to the larynx like 'karate' blow or in an accidental fall on front of neck on the handle bar of a bicycle can cause a fracture in its midline, more so, when the thyroid cartilage is calcified in an elderly aged. Thyroid cartilage when ossified may be broken into multiple fragments on application of pressure by foot. The cricoid cartilage is broken on its sides in throttling due to calcium deposits in elderly aged.

FRACTURE OF CLAVICLE

The collar bone is vulnerable in criminal assaults and accidental falls, being subcutaneous. It is placed nearly horizontal across the anterior part of root of neck. Blows causing localized impacts from blunt weapons like a stick (lathi), iron rod or a heavy stone, which can break the bone (Fig. 14.4). The fracture line is commonly transverse across the long axis of the collar bone and mostly it is in its middle third. The nature of fracture is a simple one in which the skin is intact and the fracture is located at the site of impact. This type of fracture is a direct one as the direct force is responsible to cause it. The broken fragments of the collar bone are displaced at the fracture site causing deformity and the shoulder is displaced downwards. Indirect fractures of the collar bone are usually oblique and occur at the junction of flattened lateral one third and the cylindrical medial two thirds, which form the weak point in the collar bone. The lateral fragment is displaced downwards due to the weight of the upper limb and the medial fragment is displaced upwards due to the pull of sternocleidomastoid muscle. At the fracture site the broken fragments form angulation of inverted 'V' with the fracture line at its angle. These accidental falls are common in falls from height and in automobile road accidents.

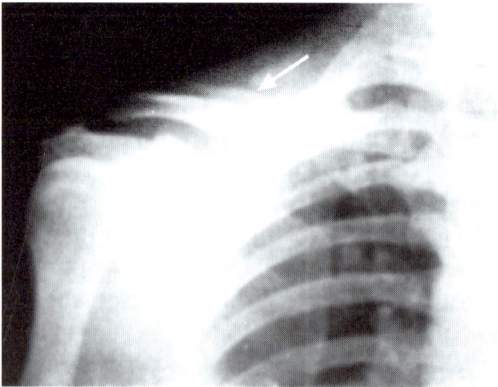

Figure 14.4: Fracture of right collar bone (indirect oblique fracture at the junction of its middle third and outer third)

The indirect oblique fracture in the collarbone occurs in accidental falls due to transmitted force from the forearm and the arm on the out stretched hand in an attempt to save oneself at the time of falling.

COMMON TRAUMATIC INJURIES AROUND THE SHOULDER JOINT

DISLOCATION OR SUBLUXATION OF STERNOCLAVICULAR JOINT

The injury to the sternoclavicular joint is caused in an accidental fall at the shoulder and also in a criminal assault by using a blunt weapon and the blunt force. Subluxation (incomplete or partial dislocation) of the sternoclavicular joint can occur in a similar situation. The inner end of the clavicle is displaced forward and upwards and can be easily seen in an X-ray film (Fig. 14.5).

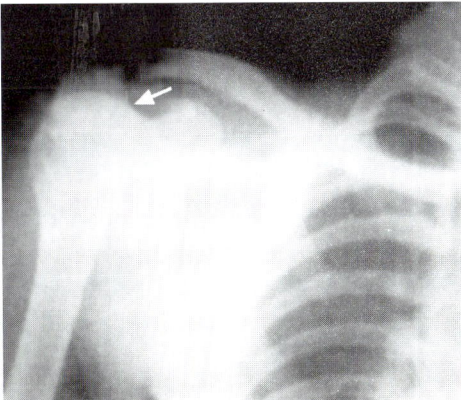

Figure 14.5: Upward and posterior dislocation of right shoulder

DISLOCATION OF ACROMIOCLAVICULAR JOINT

The injury to the acromioclavicular joint can occur due to an inflicted injury or in a fall of heavy weight (in weight lifters) on the point of shoulder, which can result in dislocation of acromioclavicular joint when violent traction is applied to the arm. It can cause complete dislocation at the joint making the outer end of the clavicle more prominent as it gets elevated.

TRAUMA TO THE SHOULDER JOINT

In criminal assaults, blunt force injuries are inflicted on the shoulder joint causing trauma to the joint and its surrounding tissues. Accidental and suicidal forceful falls often result in injury to the shoulder joint; commonly occurs in the adult. Heavy weights falling on the shoulder joint cause shoulder dislocation and fracture of neck of humerus. The greater tuberosity of the proximal end of humerus also may be forcibly separated in these injuries. Anterior dislocations of the shoulder joints also occur commonly.

DISLOCATION OF THE SHOULDER JOINT

THE ANTERIOR DISLOCATION OF THE SHOULDER JOINT

The anterior dislocation of the shoulder joint shows the head of humerus dislocated and placed below the coracoid process (i.e. subcoracoid dislocation). The head of humerus may occupy the position below the clavicle (i.e. subglenoid dislocation).

POSTERIOR DISLOCATION OF THE SHOULDER JOINT

The posterior dislocation of the shoulder joints is rare. When present it is difficult to visualize in the X-ray film. The head of the humerus usually occupies the position below the acromion process (i.e. subacrominal dislocation).

FRACTURE OF NECK OF THE HUMERUS

Fracture of anatomical neck and surgical neck of humerus are common due to blunt force injuries and their impacts on the shoulder joint. The direct fractures occur at the surgical neck commonly than at anatomical neck. Transmitted force in a fall on the outstretched hand caused indirect fracture of the anatomical neck of humerus, which is intracapsular. In these two types of fractures the broken ends are irregular and get impacted in most of the cases. Their shafts are seen abducted in both the fractures (i.e. anatomical neck and that of the surgical neck of humerus).

FRACTURES OF THE SHAFT OF THE HUMERUS

A simple fracture in the shaft of humerus is due to an accidental fall and localized impact. The fracture may be transverse, oblique or spiral. It may occur due to direct bending force or indirect transmitted twisting force and violence from a blow inflicted by a blunt weapon in a criminal assault. The fracture in the shaft of humerus is mostly comminuted (Figs 14.6 and 14.7).

INJURIES OF THE ELBOW

In injuries to the elbow, dislocations and fractures of the distal end of humerus take place giving rise to local deformity.

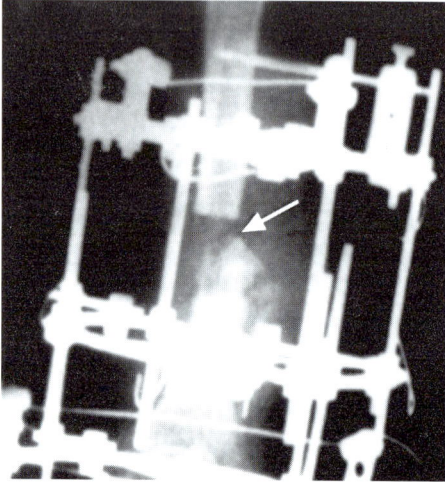

Figure 14.6: Comminuted fracture in the shaft of humerus (at the junction of its upper two thirds and the lower one third treated by external fixation)

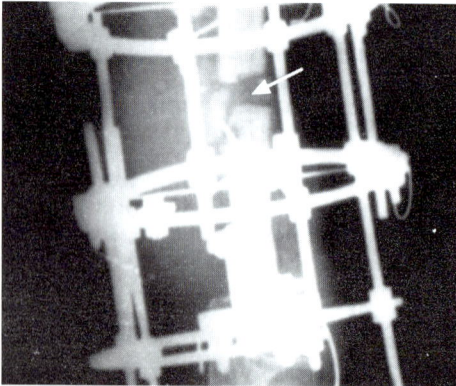

Figure 14.7: Comminuted fracture in the shaft of humerus (The same X-ray in a different view)

DISLOCATION OF THE ELBOW

In adults, the posterior dislocation is common. The proximal ends of the ulna and radius are seen displaced posteriorly. In such fractures, the elbow occupies the position of flexion. The olecranon process of ulna becomes more prominent posteriorly in the elbow. The lateral and anteroposterior view radiographs of the elbow joint are the best views to demonstrate the dislocations and fractures around the elbow joint.

FRACTURES OF THE DISTAL END OF THE HUMERUS

These are due to fall on outstretched hand when the elbow is slightly flexed. The fracture line usually involves the growth plate of cartilage.

The Supracondylar Fractures

The supracondylar fractures are most common in children. The lower fragment is displaced backwards, upwards and tilted outwards. In flexion type of supracondylar fracture the distal fragment is displaced forwards. Anteroposterior views of the X-ray reveals the fracture line place transversely just above the medial condyle of the humerus. In lateral view, the fracture line runs upwards and backwards. The fracture separation of the medial and lateral condyle of the humerus occurs in children and the young before the complete fusion with the shaft. In the X-ray the fragment of lateral condyle is seen pulled downwards and rotated. 'T' and 'Y' shaped fractures of the lower end of humerus in adults are due to violent falls on the point of elbow. These are intercondylar fractures of the lower end of humerus. In reading an X-ray film the presence of epiphyseal line is often wrongly diagnosed as the fracture line at the lower end of the humerus.

DISLOCATION AND SUBLUXATION OF THE HEAD OF RADIUS

The dislocation and subluxation of the head of radius occurs commonly in children due to pull of their forearms. Epiphyseal separation of head of radius and fracture of head and neck of the radius are common in children due to fall on the outstretched hand.

FRACTURES OF THE PROXIMAL END OF THE RADIUS

The radial head may be fractured vertically but rare. The fractured head of the radius when isolated from its shaft mostly gets tilted forwards and outwards showing distortion locally. The fracture dislocation of the head of radius may be associated with the fracture of upper third of ulna with the radial head displaced anteriorly (Monteggia fracture). It is possible to sustain a reversed 'Monteggia' fracture with the radial head dislocated posteriorly and the ulnar fracture displaced posteriorly.

FRACTURE OF THE PROXIMAL END OF ULNA

The fracture of the proximal end of ulna from a direct fall on the back of elbow. The fracture line is located at the junction of the olecranon process and the shaft of ulna. Fractures of upper third of ulna occurs in "Monteggia" fracture dislocation, which occurs commonly in adults.

FRACTURE OF THE MIDDLE THIRD OF SHAFT OF ULNA

The fracture of middle third of shaft of ulna occurs in combination with fracture in the middle third of the radius due to localized impacts from blunt weapons in criminal assaults. These fractures are horizontal or oblique and reveal displacement and overlapping rarely, the fracture may occur in radius alone or in ulna alone and that possibility exists in accidental falls and in criminal assaults.

Fracture of ulna and radius in children are accidental due to fall and the fractures are often 'green-stick' fractures (Fig. 14.8).

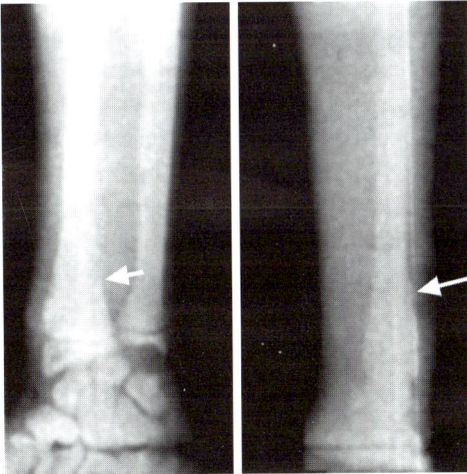

Figure 14.8: Green-stick fracture in distal one third of right radius

FRACTURE DISLOCATIONS OF THE DISTAL END OF THE RADIUS

Fracture dislocation of the distal end of the radius occurs in children when the epiphysis of the distal end of the radius is not united to the shaft completely. The fracture in the distal third of shaft of radius occurs with fracture dislocation of lower end of radius in association with distal radioulnar joint dislocation (Galaezzi fracture dislocation), which occurs commonly in a fall on the ground with rotational forces as seen in automobile accidents. The fracture of distal end of radius giving rise to 'dinner fork deformity', i.e. Colles fracture, with displacement of the distal fragment proximal and posteriorly with rotation and little radial deviation is caused by a fall on the heel of palm firmly coming in contact with the ground. On X-ray examination the fractured distal end of radius is seen displaced backwards, upwards and laterally. The fracture line is usually one inch (2.5 cm) above the wrist joint and the styloid process of ulna and the styloid process of radius lie at the same level in the X-ray. The Colle's fracture may be associated with the fracture of styloid process of ulna also. The reverse Colles' fracture is the "Smith's Fracture", which is less common and occurs due to a fall on the dorsum of the hand when the wrist joint is flexed (Figs 14.9 to 14.11). In Smith's fracture the distal fragment is anteriorly displaced with slight rotation.

DISLOCATION AND FRACTURES OF CARPAL BONES

1. Dislocation of lunate occurs in a fall on the dorsiflexed hand due to hyperextension. In X-ray

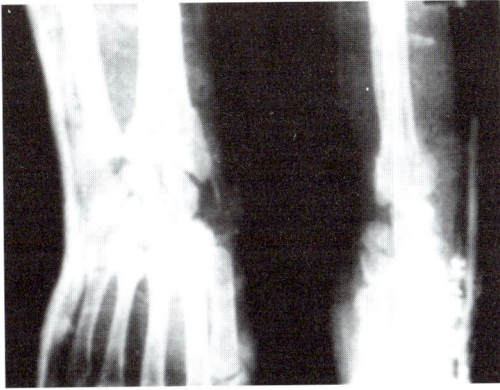

Figure 14.9: Colles' fractures of right hand (after reduction and POP)

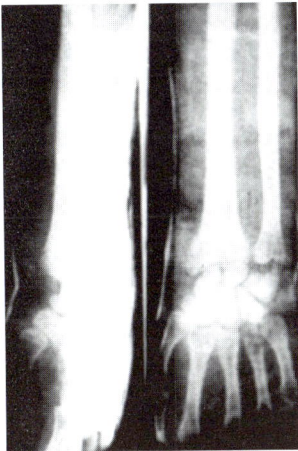

Figure 14.10: Fractures of right radius with fractures of styloid process of right ulna

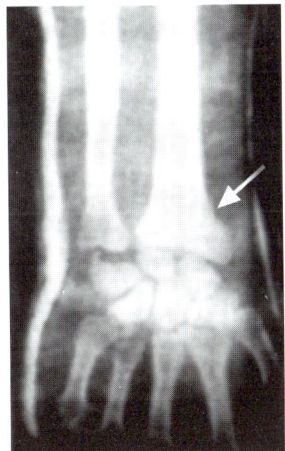

Figure 14.11: Colles' fracture with fracture lines and POP, after reduction

lateral view of the wrist, the lunate is seen dislocated anteriorly.

2. Fracture of the scaphoid occurs in an accidental fall and fracture line involves the narrowed mid region of the scaphoid bone, which can be viewed in the oblique view of the X-ray only. Anteroposterior and lateral views do not detect the fracture line. The fracture site becomes more radiolucent in a weeks period due to bone resorption. Bony union is delayed and often ends in nonunion. The proximal fragment of the broken scaphoid shows avascular necrosis.

FRACTURE DISLOCATION OF METACARPAL BONES OF THE HAND (FIGS 14.12 AND 14.13)

FRACTURE DISLOCATION AT THE BASE OF FIRST METACARPAL BONE

Fracture dislocation at the base of first metacarpal bone is known as 'Bennets' fracture dislocation' and the fracture site reveals prominence of the base of first metacarpal bone.

FRACTURES OF THE SHAFTS OF METACARPAL BONES

These fractures occur due to direct violence in criminal assaults using blunt weapons on the victim and are known as 'defence injuries' sustained in defending himself. Theses fractures present abnormal bony projections with loss of alignment of the knuckles and reveal irregular fractured ends.

FRACTURES OF PHALANGES

These fractures occur in criminal assaults by direct violence. They reveal local deformity and irregular broken ends.

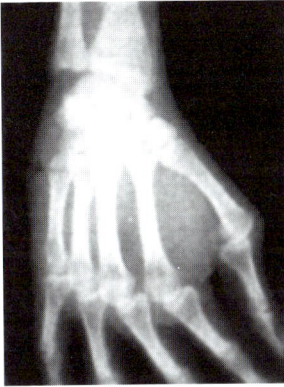

Figure 14.12: Fracture base of fifth metacarpal bone

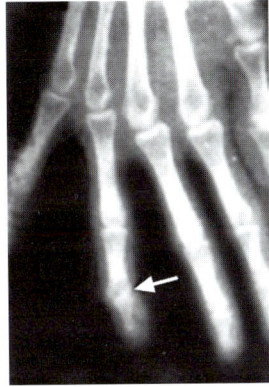

Figure 14.13: Fracture middle phalanx of right ring finger

DISLOCATION OF METACARPOPHALANGEAL JOINTS AND INTERPHALANGEAL JOINTS

These injuries occur due to hyperextension. They reveal excess prominence of the heads dorsally.

DISLOCATIONS AND FRACTURES OF CERVICAL VERTEBRAE

Dislocations and fractures of cervical vertebrae result from direct violence and indirect violence. They are caused commonly from intense forcible bending (hyperflexion) occurring in a fall and landing on buttocks or on the feet. The upper and lower cervical vertebrae (CV) are involved in the neck (Figs 14.14 and 14.15). Dislocations usually occur between the fourth and the fifth CV or the fifth and sixth CV in a fall from height and also from falling of heavy

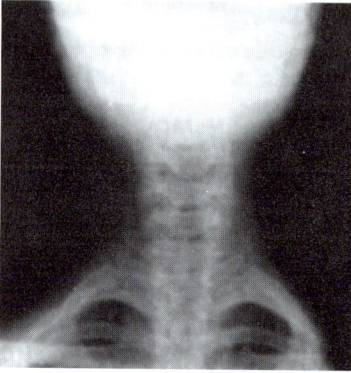

Figure 14.14: Anteroposterior radiograph of neck showing cervical vertebrae

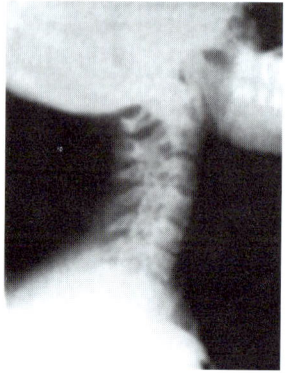

Figure 14.15: Lateral radiograph of neck showing cervical vertebrae

weights on the back result in fracture – dislocations of the cervical vertebrae. In traffic accidents, the driver and the front seat occupants sustain fracture dislocation of cervical vertebrae due to sudden hyperflexion and hyperextension by the forces of acceleration and deceleration. These injuries are termed 'whiplash' injuries caused in vehicular accidents due to sudden stop or in a collision. A forceful blow on the neck from a blunt weapon also may cause such injuries to the cervical vertebrae. Hyperextension often causes forward dislocation of the odontoid process of the second cervical vertebra resulting in death. Transverse fracture of odontoid process occurs at its base and it occurs in hyperflexion and hyperextension injuries to the neck. In judicial hanging, dislocation occurs between the atlas and the axis.

FRACTURES OF THE SPINOUS PROCESSES, TRANSVERSE PROCESSES, LAMINAE AND PEDICLES

These injuries are caused in flexion and extension of the spinal column.

DISLOCATION AND FRACTURES OF THORACIC AND LUMBAR VERTEBRAE

Forcible bending at the junction of the thoracic and lumbar vertebrae results in 'compression' type of fractures in vertebral bodies. The bodies of thoracic and lumbar vertebrae are spongy and fragile. They are crushed into 'wedge' shaped vertebral bodies seen in lateral views of the X-rays taken (Figs 14.16 and 14.17).

THORAX AND ABDOMEN

Posteroanterior chest X-ray shows images of bones of the chest wall and of the soft tissues.

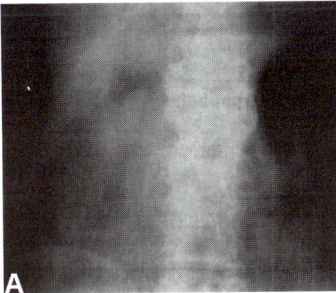

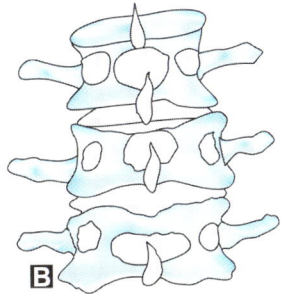

Figures 14.16A and B: (A) Compression fracture of first lumbar vertebra (AP view); (B) Lumbar vertebrae

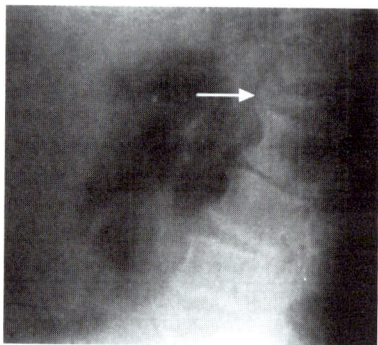

Figure 14.17: Compression fracture of first lumbar vertebra (lateral view)

A. Images of bones of the chest wall (Fig. 14.3A)
  1. Clavicles (right and left).
  2. Ribs (bilateral and symmetrical).
  3. Thoracic vertebral part of the spinal column.
  4. Scapulae (right and left).
B. Images of the soft tissues of the thorax
  1. Dooms of the diaphragm (right and left).
  2. Fundus of the stomach with gas/air.
  3. Cardiovascular shadows.
  4. Lungs (right and left) with their lung fields, bronchial markings and their hilum.

Clavicles

The clavicles are fractured by direct and indirect force. The fracture line may be transverse or oblique at the junction of inner two-thirds and the outer one-third. The fracture site is mostly angulated.

Ribs

The ribs are fractured in criminal assaults. Severe fist blows are inflicted on the chest. Kicks and blows from blunt weapons also cause rib fractures. Usually one or two ribs are fractured due to localized impacts. The jagged, sharp broken ends are directed inwards. These are direct injuries inflicted to the chest wall. The indirect rib fractures result from impacts in falls from height due to transmitted force. The middle ribs from fourth to eighth are fractured commonly in midaxillary line and in the line of angles of the ribs by indirect transmitted force. Comminuted fractures of ribs result in run-over vehicular and bullock-cart accidents. Falling of heavy weights in collapse of buildings, the rafter, boulders and debris causes comminuted fracture of ribs. In criminal violence using pressure by the knees over the chest often results in bilateral symmetrical fractures both in front and back of the chest, mostly near the costo-chondral junctions anteriorly and at the angles of the ribs posteriorly. There may be associated transverse "buckle" fracture of the sternum.

Thoracic Vertebrae

The vertebral bodies of thoracic vertebrae being spongy are compressed into wedge-shapes in accidental falls from heights and from falling of heavy weights on back causing severe bending and crushing of the vertebral bodies.

Scapula

Fractures of scapula are mostly due to direct trauma but they are rare.

IMAGES OF SOFT TISSUE SHADOWS SHOWING ABNORMAL FINDINGS

1. Both the dooms of the diaphragm are flattened in long standing asthma and emphysema.
2. Unilateral or bilateral blunting of the costophrenic angles indicate pleural effusion.
3. Presence of gas under the dooms of diaphragm indicates perforation or rupture of the hollow viscera in the abdominal cavity (pneumoperitoneum).
   The gas accumulation under the diaphragm produces a radiolucent area in the skiagram.
4. Stomach is indicated beneath the left doom of the diaphragm from the presence of air, which produces radiolucent area.
5. Cardiovascular area: In a skiagram it may indicate enlargement or distortion.

PLAIN X-RAY OF ABDOMEN

A plain X-ray of abdomen when taken shows bony pelvis, lower thoracic vertebrae. Lower ribs, five lumbar vertebrae.

BONY PELVIS

In accidental falls from height and in traffic accidents the bony pelvis sustains fractures in hip-bones and fracture dislocation in sacroiliac joints and in symphysis pubis.

LOWER-THORACIC VERTEBRAE AND LOWER RIBS

The plain X-ray of abdomen shows lower two or three thoracic vertebrae and 11th and 12th ribs. The thoracic vertebrae present their concave sides in their bodies and transverse processes extending laterally; their spinous process in the midline project beyond their lower border and present 'tear-drop' appearance. The pedicles on lateral part in each vertebra appear elliptical in outline.

LUMBAR VERTEBRA

The five lumbar vertebrae are seen in the plain X-ray of abdomen. The body of each lumbar vertebra appears rectangular and shows concave sides. Their pedicles present elliptical outlines and spinous processes shows tear-drop outlines and project below and lower border in midline.

OTHER PARTS OF THE PELVIS

Pelvis Inlet

The pelvic inlet presents its shape and indicates the sex. In a male it is heart shaped, triangular (android type) and in female it is rounded (circular/gynecoid type).

Sub-pubic Angle

The sub-pubic angle in a male is narrow inverted V-shaped and less than 90° and whereas in female it is wider, inverted U-shaped and more than 90°.

Sacrum and Coccyx

Sacrum is longer and narrower in the male and short and wider in the female. As the sacrum is formed by fusion of five vertebrae, its pelvic surface shows four transverse ridges at their site of fusion. The pelvic surface shows four pelvic sacral foramen on either side.

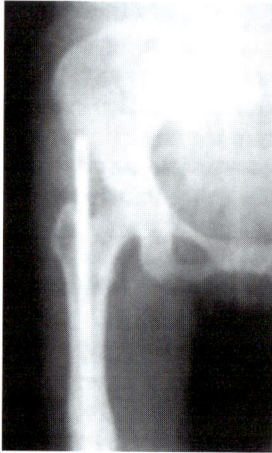

Figure 14.18: United fracture/healed fracture with callous formation (intramedullary nailing in fracture of femur)

Coccyx

The coccyx is triangular in shape and consists of four rudimentary vertebrae fused together. It is united at the sacro-coccygeal joint with cartilaginous disk and the ligaments (Fig. 14.18).

COMMON TRAUMATIC INJURIES OF THE BONY PELVIS AND ITS JOINTS

Fractures of the pelvis are common in road accidents as a result of forcible fall against the hard surface of the ground or in primary impact. The injuries to the bony pelvis are mostly due to run over accidents caused by heavy vehicles like trucks and loaded lorries. A forcible fall from a great height also often results in pelvis fractures.

THE PUBIC RAMII

The superior and inferior ramus are commonly fractured and reveal bony discontinuity with irregular ends of the broken bone.

THE SYMPHYSIS PUBIS

The pubic symphysis gets dislocated in traffic accidents and railway run-over accidents. The fracture dislocation of symphysis pubis also occurs due to fall of a heavy weight on the point of symphysis pubis resulting in gross displacement of the pubic bones on either side.

THE SACROILIAC JOINTS

These joints are often dislocated in falls from height, in road traffic accidents and in accidental railway run over injuries.

DISLOCATION OF THE HIP JOINT

Trauma to the hip joint causes its dislocation. It may be a posterior dislocation or an anterior dislocation and rarely the central dislocation.

POSTERIOR DISLOCATION

The posterior dislocation of the femoral head from its articulation in the acetabulum is most common. The head of femur is displaced upwards (superior) from the socket of acetabulum. The shaft of the femur assumes an adducted position and internal rotation. The X-ray taken reveals the head of femur outside the socket of acetabulum and is placed above it.

ANTERIOR DISLOCATION

The anterior dislocation of the femoral head from its articulation in the acetabulum and the head of femur is displaced downwards (inferiorly) from the cavity of acetabulum. The shaft of the femur appears abducted and externally rotated. The X-ray taken reveals the head of femur outside the acetabular cavity and placed below it.

CENTRAL DISLOCATION

Fractures of acetabulum occur when the head of femur is forced through its socket in vehicular collision accidents. The driver sustains the injury in his hip-joint, known as 'dash-board' injury. This type of injury causes discontinuity in the Shenton's line. In anterior and posterior dislocations of the femoral head from the socket of acetabulum also causes deformed outline or discontinuity in the Shenton's line.

FRACTURE OF THE NECK OF FEMUR

Fracture of the neck of femur occurs in a young individual in a forcible injury to the hip-joint. In an elderly individual a minor fall on the hip causes a pathological fracture due to osteoporosis and rarefaction in the neck of femur. In fracture of the neck of femur the fracture line may be in the upper third or in the lower part of the neck of femur (Fig. 14.19). These fractures in the middle part are "transcervical"; in the trochanter are "subtrochanteric". The fractured ends in these fractures are mostly impacted.

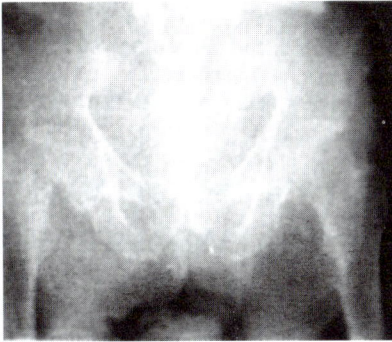

Figure 14.19: Fracture neck of right femur in its upper third (sub: Capital fracture)

FRACTURES OF THE SHAFT OF THE FEMUR

The femur is broken in severe trauma being a strong bone in the body. Local bleeding inside the thigh is severe and causes shock. The direct violence is necessary to cause the fracture in the shaft. The fracture in the shaft may involve the upper third, middle third or the lower third. When the fracture is in the upper third of femoral shaft, the proximal fragment gets displaced medially and shows over riding and outward angulation. In fractures of lower third of the shaft the distal fragment is seen flexed.

COMMON TRAUMATIC INJURIES OF THE KNEE

Severe injuries to the knee result in fractures of patella and fracture of distal end of femur and the proximal end of tibia.

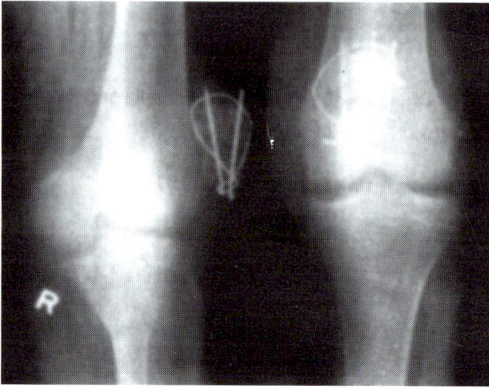

Figure 14.20: Comminuted fracture of the patella (showing surgical wiring)—lateral view and AP view

FRACTURE OF THE PATELLA (Fig. 14.20)

The patellar fractures are caused from direct blunt force impacts on the anterior aspect of the knee either accidental or intentional in criminal assaults. Transverse fractures of patella are common. A forcible direct injury to the knee-cap can cause "comminuted fracture", the patella breaking into multiple fragments. The transverse fracture of patella reveals a gap between the two broken fragments due to proximal and distal retraction. Forcible active contraction of the strong quadriceps femoris muscle break the bone transversely into, two fragments which are pulled apart. The transverse fracture mostly involve the entire thickness of the bone.

FRACTURES OF DISTAL END OF FEMUR AND THE PROXIMAL END OF TIBIA

In 'hit and run' heavy vehicular accidents, a pedestrian is commonly knocked down from his standing position and sustains direct severe injury to the knee. The injury may be unilateral or bilateral and symmetrical produced by the forcible contact (i.e., primary impact injuries) of the 'bumper' (fender) of the heavy vehicle like a lorry or a truck. The injury about the knee is mostly intracapsular.

FRACTURE OF THE TIBIA AND FIBULA

The tibia is weight bearing and subcutaneous (most of its shaft in its anteromedial surface) and is vulnerable for direct injuries resulting in fractures. The fractures in the shaft of tibia are mostly in traffic accidents and in falls from height. Both the bones of the legs are fractured mostly at the same level. In falls the lower third of the tibia is mostly fractured (Figs 14.21A and B). Isolated injury to the fibula is rare.

The fractures of tibia are often open or compound fractures being subcutaneous. Anteroposterior and lateral views of the X-rays reveal the type of fracture. They may be transverse, oblique, spiral and comminuted and often show overriding of the broken fragments. A depressed fracture in the lateral condyle of the tibia in its proximal end is caused from a forcible hit and is intracapsular.

COMMON TRAUMATIC INJURIES ABOUT THE ANKLE JOINT

The common injuries are fractures and fracture dislocations of the ankle.

ABDUCTION FRACTURES

Transverse fracture of fibula and fracture of medial malleolus commonly occurs due to forceful abduction

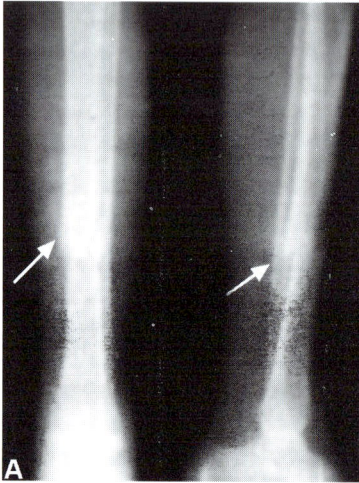

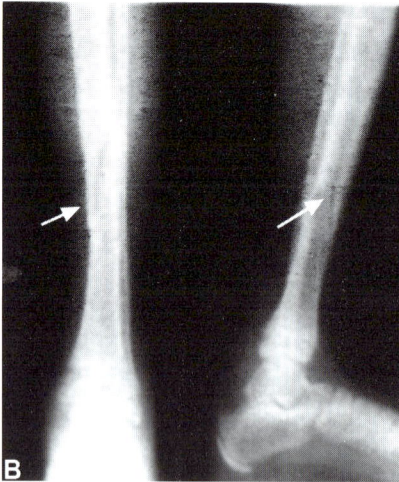

Figures 14.21A and B: Fracture lower third of
left tibia—AP and lateral views

force acting on the ankle joint and the foot is forcibly abducted. The fibula is fractured transverse in nearly two inches (5 cm) above the ankle joint.

ADDUCTION FRACTURES

The adduction force acting on the ankle also causes transverse fracture of the lateral malleolus and vertical fracture in the medial malleolus.

EXTERNAL ROTATION FRACTURES

Twisting force acting on the ankle with the foot resting on the ground causes fracture of the distal end of fibula and transverse fracture of medial malleolus. External rotation injury of the ankle results in oblique fracture of lateral malleolus, i.e. distal end of fibula.

Anteroposterior: Lateral (Fig. 14.22) and oblique views of X-rays are useful in the examination of ankle joint injuries.

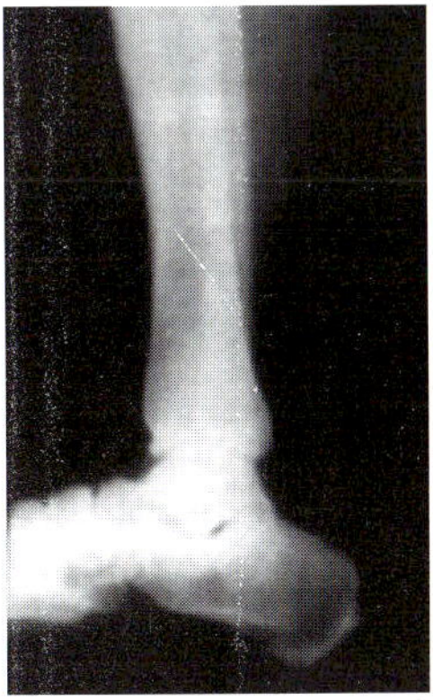

Figure 14.22: Fracture of medial malleolus of right tibia (in its distal end)—lateral view

FRACTURES OF THE CALCANEUM

The injury to the calcaneum is mostly compression type of fracture. It results due to a fall from a great height (nearly 100 feet) and landing on foot. Both the ankles and feet are commonly injured. Mostly these injuries are common in the adults.

FRACTURES OF THE TALUS

The fractures are caused to the talus in a fall on the feet with the dorsiflexion. The displacement of the fragments is common in fractures of the talus.

INJURIES OF THE METATARSALS AND PHALANGES OF THE FOOT (FIGS 14.23 TO 14.25)

1. Avulsion fractures of the base of fifth metatarsal bone (Jones' fractures): These fractures occur due to forceful inversion of the foot. The fracture line is either

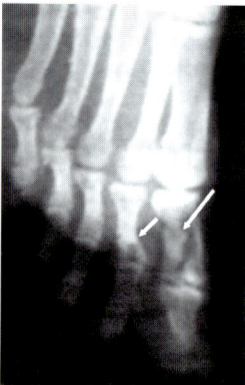

Figure 14.23: Fracture of proximal phalanx of big toe and second toe of right foot

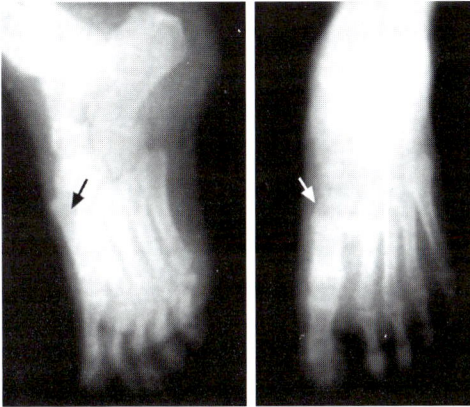

Figure 14.24: Fracture dislocation of proximal end of left first metatarsal bone of foot

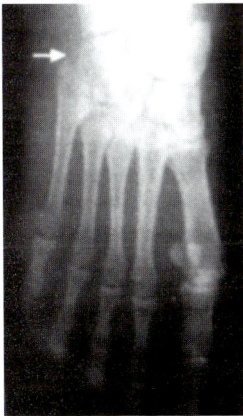

Figure 14.25: Fracture base of left fifth metatarsal bone of foot

transverse or oblique passing through the base of the fifth metatarsal.

2. Other injuries to the foot occur from direct violence. Heavy weights falling directly on the feet cause crushing injuries.

3

Other Cases of Medicolegal Importance

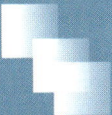

Chapter 15

Other Cases of Medicolegal Importance

Anteroposterior radiograph (Fig. 15.1) of the lungs removed after postmortem examination shows distended appearance of lungs due to pulmonary edema (a lock-up death).

Lobes of lung are cut into number of pieces and examined for tuberculosis lesions, if any.

Acute left ventricular failure and sudden death may result in a young individual suffering from essential

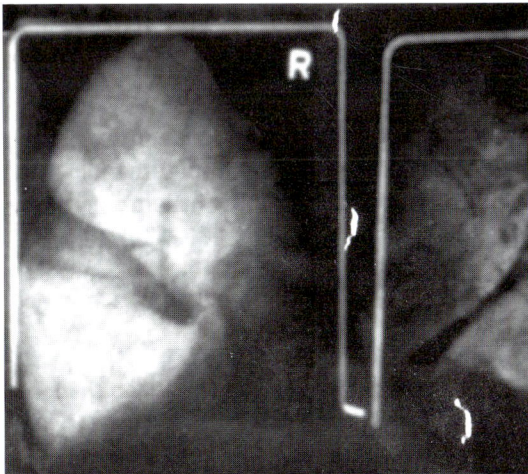

Figure 15.1: Anteroposterior radiograph

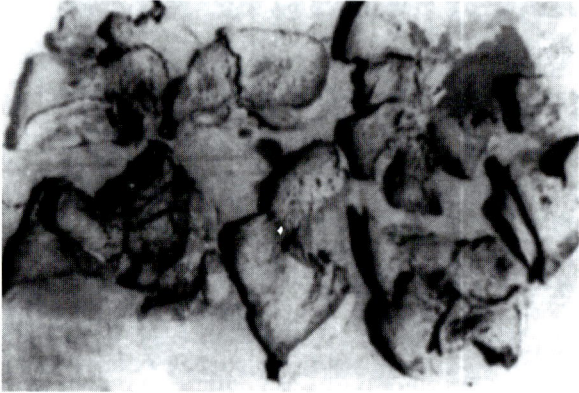

Figure 15.2: No tuberculous lesions in cut lung pieces. Alveolar spaces are filled with edema fluid

hypertension. Edematous lungs are heavy and moist on gross examination in postmortem examination. Cut surface of lungs exudes frothy blood (Fig. 15.2). Microscopic examination shows congestion of alveolar capillaries in their septa and the alveolar spaces are filled with edema fluid (pink proteinaceous material with RBCs and macrophages).

On examination of the heart: It shows increase in weight more than 500 g, thickness of left ventricle more than 15 mm and the lumen of left ventricle is smaller. These changes are due to concentric hypertrophy of the myocardium of the heart.

On microscopic examination each cardiac muscle fiber revealed increase in size with foci of degeneration and necrosis.

Electron Microscopy: Reveals increase in myofibrils and changes in mitochondria. RNA is increased and ratio of

RNA to DNA is also increased in myocardial fibers, which are hypertrophied (Pulmonary tuberculosis was alleged by the IO being a lockup death. But the lungs revealed only pulmonary edema and to tubercular lesions. Histopathology of tissue did not reveal any tuberculosis).

FINDINGS IN A TYPICAL CASE OF TB LUNGS

Tubercular lesions are aggregations of epithelioid cells, which form granulomas with central necrosis and multinucleated giant cells arranged in horse-shoe shapes. A zone of lymphocytes, plasma cells and fibroblasts are found at the periphery of granuloma. The central caseous material is cheesy due to its lipoid content. In advanced stage of TB, lung cavitations with fibrosis and fibrocaseous lesions are found. The caseous material may produce pneumonic consolidation in lobes.

X-RAY EXAMINATION

Shows opaque shadows of tuberculous lesions and cavitations. In military tuberculosis in acute stage show small granulomas (1 mm in diameter) disseminated all over the lung fields and reveal 'snow-storm' appearance in the X-ray.

CHOKING

Choking in children is mostly accidental. Children are in habit of placing small objects like pins, safety pins, coins, marbles and seeds in the their mouth. These objects often accidentally slip in to their larynx and get lodged, mostly above the vocal cords. They obstruct completely or partially the upper respiratory tract. Mere presence of

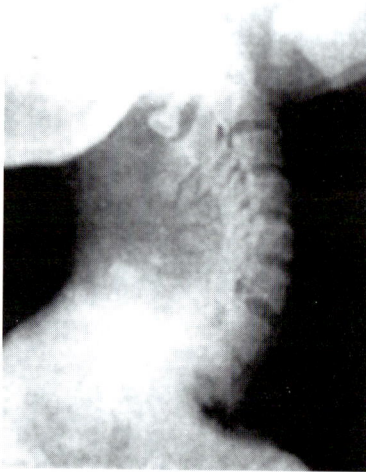

Figure 15.3: Lateral radiograph of the neck showing upper respiratory tract: Larynx and trachea. A metal pin is seen in the larynx with the sharp end directed posteriorly

foreign body stimulates vagus nerve endings (parasympathetic nerve fibers) supplying the mucous lining of the larynx (Fig. 15.3). A small flying particle of thermocol inhaled into the upper respiratory tract and the larynx can cause laryngeal spasm, respiratory distress and reflex cardiac inhibition, unconsciousness and sudden death from stimulation of vagus nerve endings. In adults, a bolus of food, a fish bone, a piece of meat, a denture and a metal pin (when used as a toothpick) for clearing food particles lodged between the teeth mostly while laughing causes choking.

4

Exercises for Age Estimation and Radiological Examinations for Sex Differences and Primary Ossification Centers of IUL

Exercises for Age Estimation and Radiological Examinations for Sex Differences and Primary Ossification Centers of IUL

. . . .

EXERCISES FOR AGE ESTIMATION (FIGS 16.1 TO 16.19)

LINE DRAWING FROM X-RAY FILM

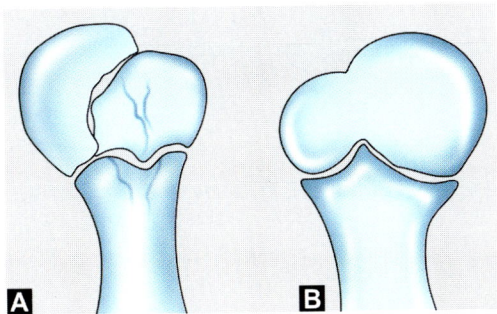

Figures 16.1A and B: Proximal ends of humerus

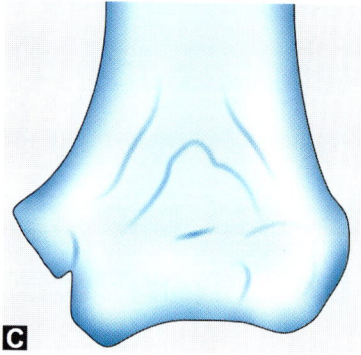

Figure 16.1C: Distal end of humerus

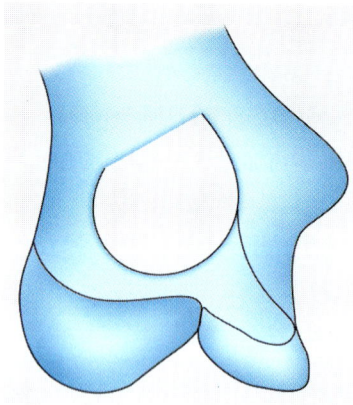

Figure 16.2: Distal end of humerus

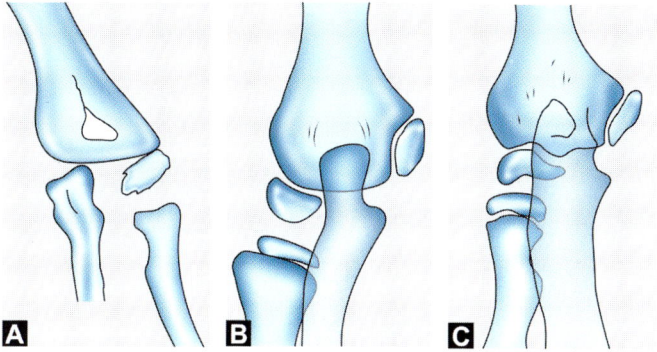

Figures 16.3A to C: Elbow joints

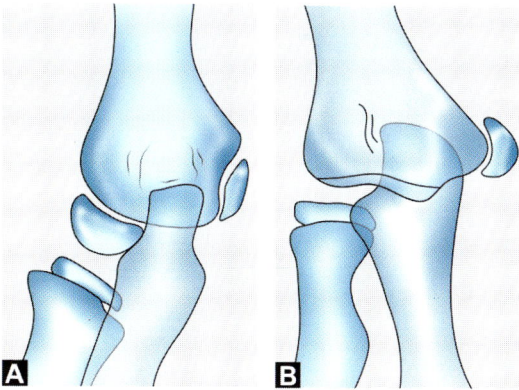

Figures 16.4A and B: Elbow joints

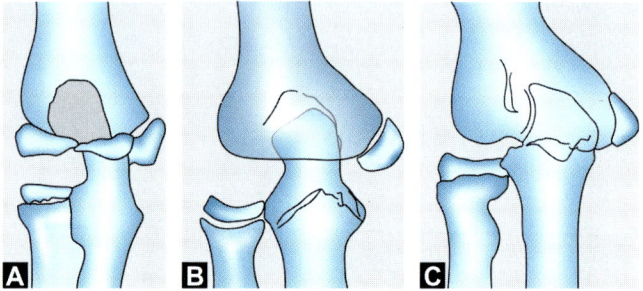

Figures 16.5A to C: Elbow joints

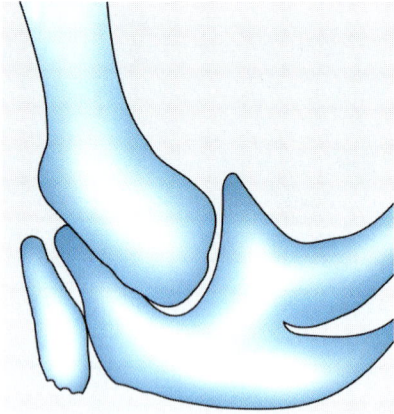

Figure 16.6: Elbow joint— lateral view

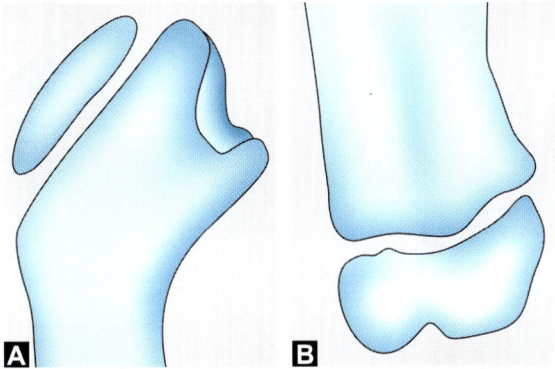

Figures 16.7A and B: (A) Proximal end of ulna;
(B) Distal end of ulna

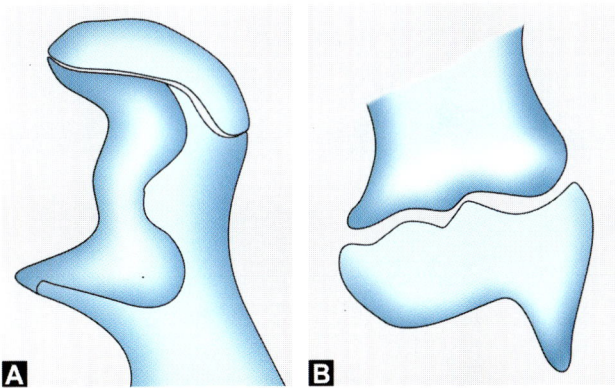

Figures 16.8A and B: (A) Proximal end of ulna;
(B) Distal end of ulna

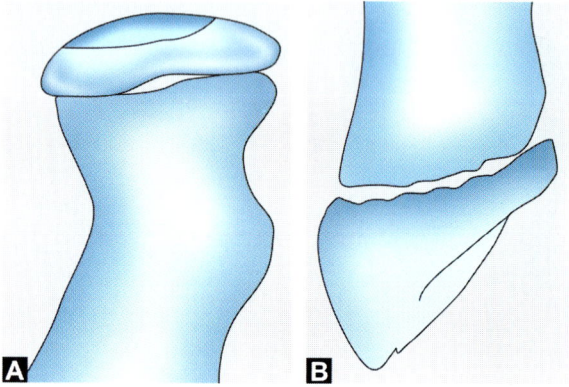

Figures 16.9A and B: (A) Proximal end of radius;
(B) Distal end of radius

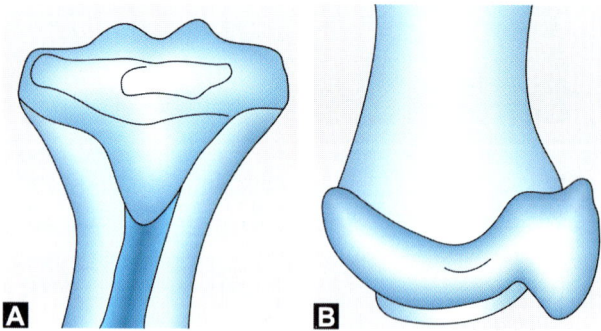

Figures 16.10A and B: (A) Proximal end of tibia;
(B) Distal end of tibia

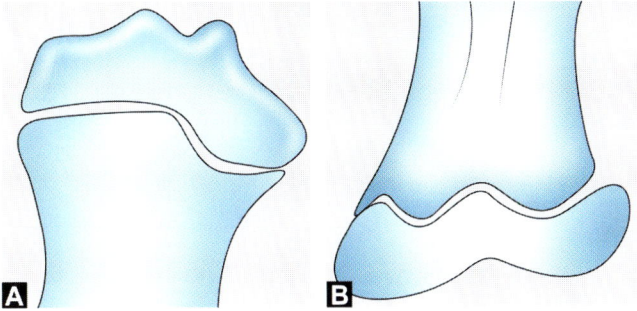

Figures 16.11A and B: (A) Proximal end of tibia;
(B) Distal end of tibia

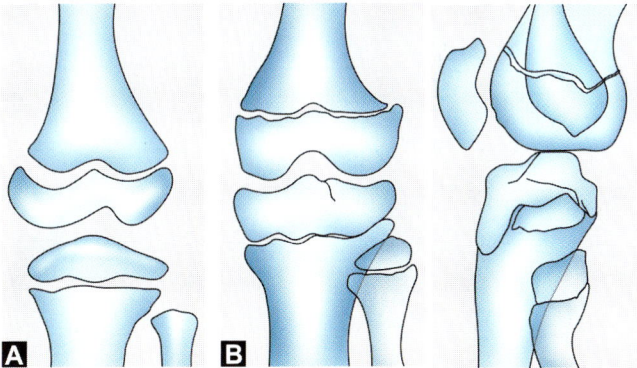

Figures 16.12A and B: (A) Knee joint;
(B) Knee joints—lateral view

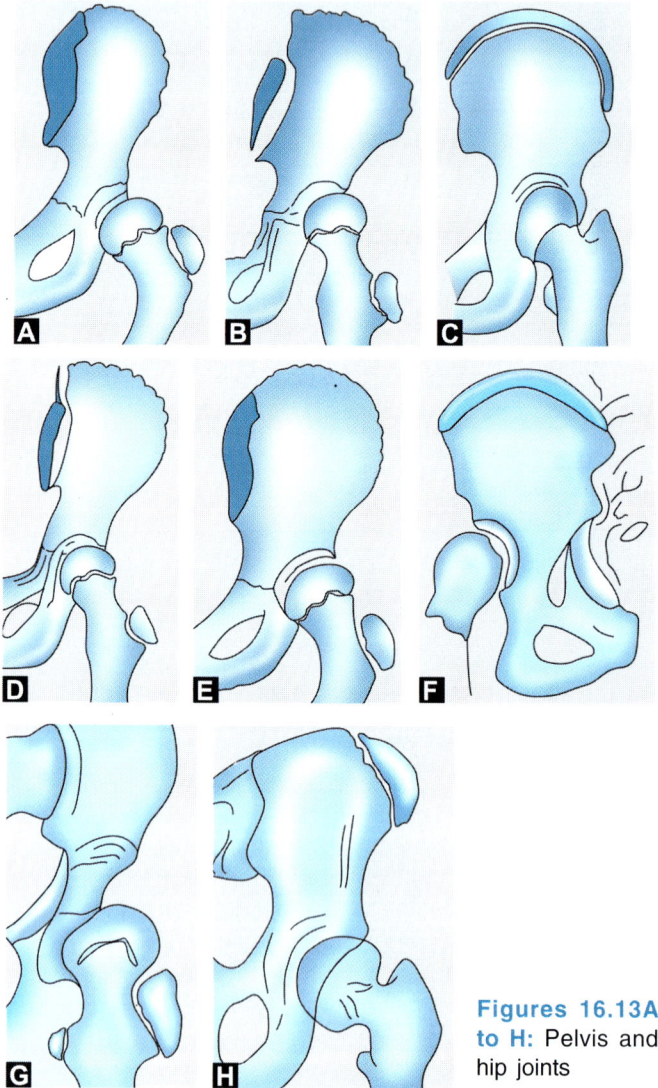

Figures 16.13A to H: Pelvis and hip joints

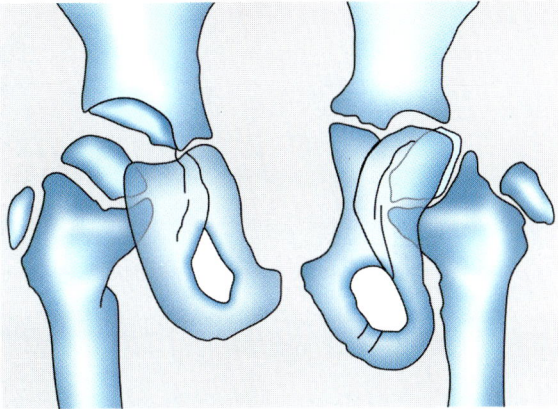

Figure 16.14: Pelvis and hip joint (child)

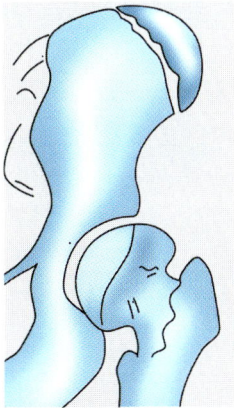

Figure 16.15: Pelvis and hip joints

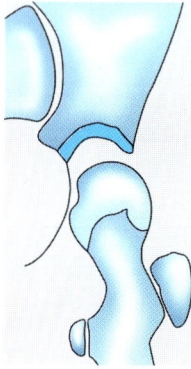

Figure 16.16: Hip joint— proximal end of femur

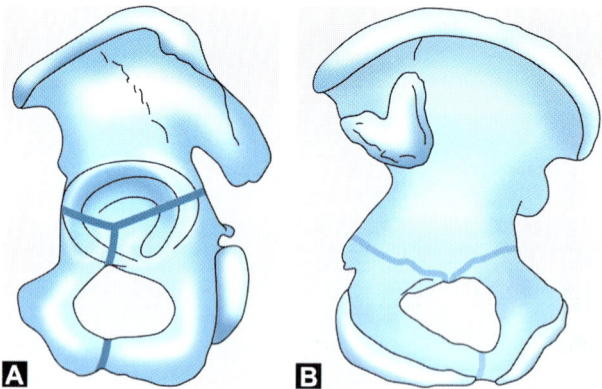

Figures 16.17A and B: Hip bones

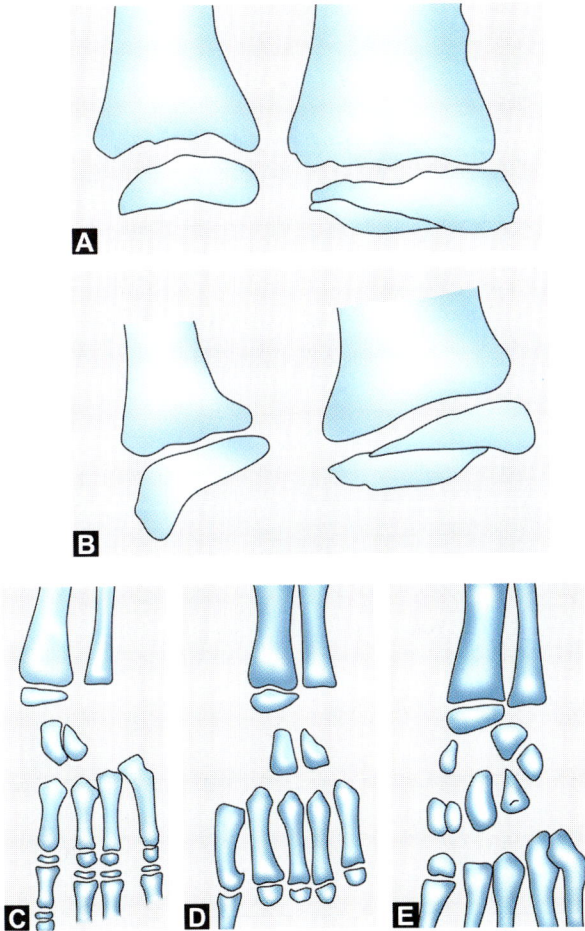

Figures 16.18A to E: Lower end of radius and ulna

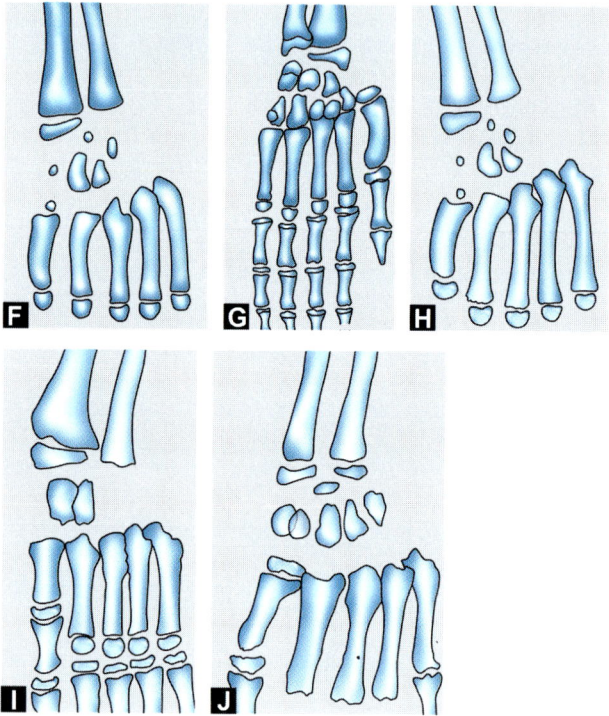

Figures 16.18F to J: Lower ends of radius and ulna

RADIOLOGICAL EXAMINATION FOR SEX DIFFERENCES IN SKULL AND PELVIS OF MALE AND FEMALE (ADULT) (FIGS 16.20 TO 16.23)

1. Skull

	Male	*Female*
• Forehead	Steeper	Vertical
• Glabella	Prominent	Not prominent
• Orbits	Square-shaped	Rounded

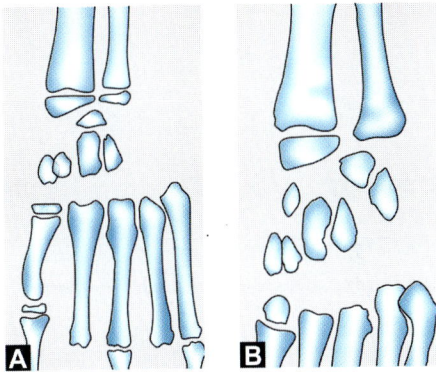

Figures 16.19A and B: Wrist, hand joint and fingers

- Supraorbital ridges   Prominent   Less prominent
- Frontal eminence   Small   Large
- Parietal eminence   Small   Large
- Occipital area
  External occipital   More marked   Less marked
  protuberance
- Mastoid process   Large   Small

2. Mandible

	Male	*Female*
Chin	Square	Rounded
Condyles	Large	Small

3. Pelvic

	Male	*Female*
Pelvic inlet (brim)	Heart shaped (Heart of playing cards) Android type	Rounded Gynecoid type

• Pelvic cavity (Cavity of true pelvis)	Funnel shaped	Broad and shallow (basin-like)
• Preauricular sulcus	Absent	Prominent deep and broad
• Acetabulum	Large	Small
• Greater sciatic notch	Deep and narrow	Shallow and wide
• Auricular surface (articular surface of sacro-iliac, articulation, i.e. auricular surface)	Large and extends to 2½ to 3 sacral vertebrae	Small and extends to 2 to 2½ sacral vertebrae
• Sacrum	Long and narrow	Short and wide

(Forward concavity more pronounced in female)

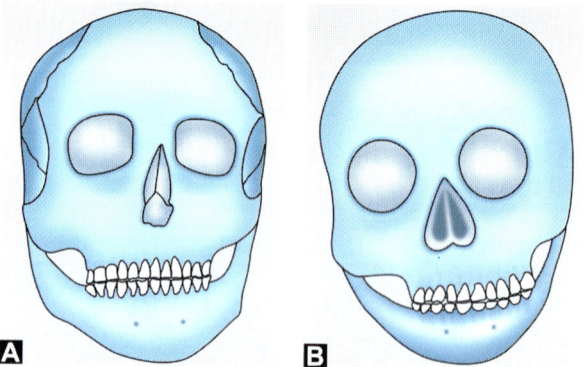

Figures 16.20A and B: (A) Male skull; (B) Female skull

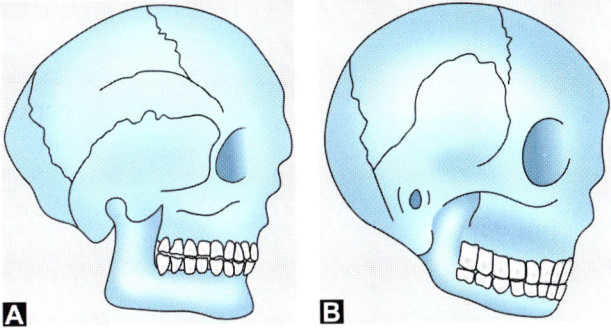

Figures 16.21A and B: (A) Male skull (lateral view);
(B) Female skull (lateral view)

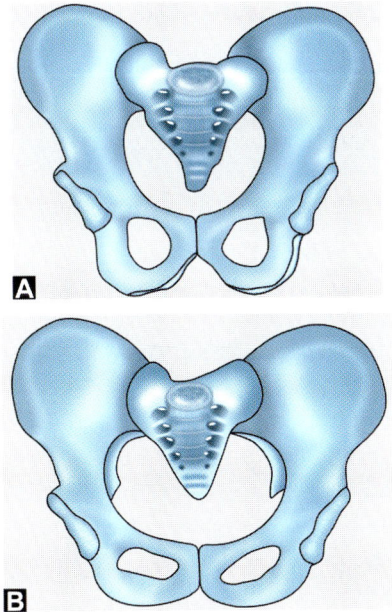

Figures 16.22A and B: (A) Male pelvis; (B) Female pelvis

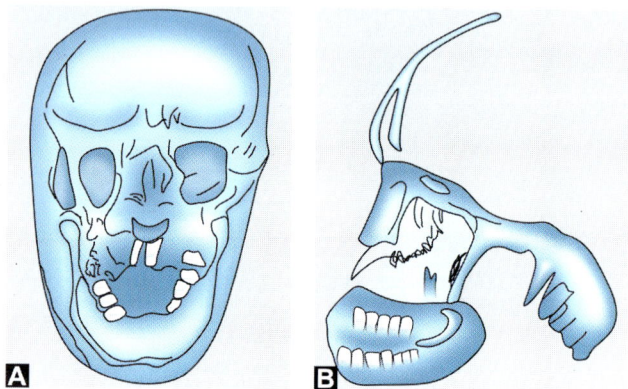

Figures 16.23A and B: (A) Skull—PA view;
(B) Face—lateral view

RADIOLOGICAL EXAMINATION FOR PRIMARY OSSIFICATION CENTERS OF INTRAUTERINE LIFE (IUL) (FIGS 16.24 TO 16.26)

1. *Cranial bones:*
   - Frontal: One
   - Parietal: Two
   - Temporal: Two
     (Ear ossicles: malleus incus and stapes)
   - Ethmoid: One
   - Sphenoid: One
   - Occipital: One
2. *Facial bones:*
   - Nasal: Two
   - Maxilla: Two
   - Zygomatic: Two
   - Palatine: Two

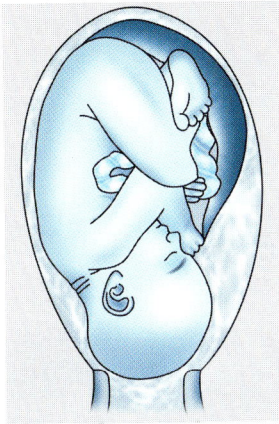

Figure 16.24: Pregnant uterus
(Full term vertex presentation)

- Lacrimal: Two
- Inferior nasal concha: Two
- Mandible: One
- Vomer: One
3. *Upper limb bones (pectoral girdle):*
   - Collar bone: Two
   - Scapula: Two
   - Humerus: Two
   - Radius and Ulna: Two (in forearm bones), each forearm.
4. *Hand and finger bones (in wrist all carpal are cartilaginous only in intrauterine life):*
   - Metacarpals: Five
   - Phalanges : Proximal
     — Middle
     — Distal

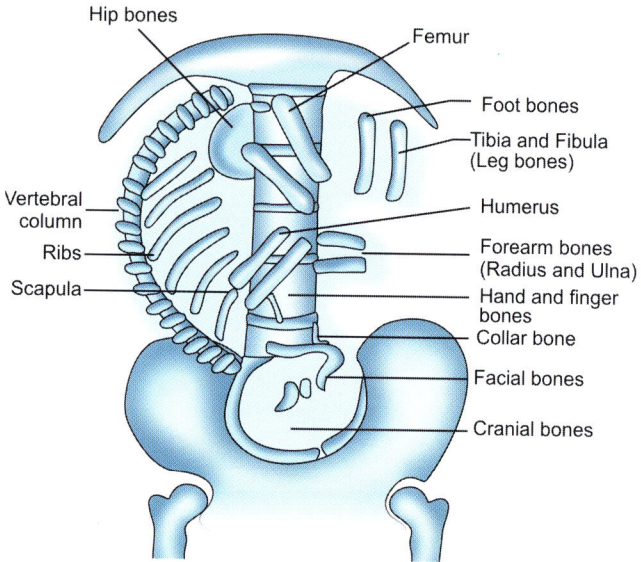

Figure 16.25: Radiological Examination for primary ossification centers in bones of fetus in intrauterine life

5. *Lower limb bones (Pelvis girdle):*
   - Hip bone: Two
     (each hip bone consists of ilium, ischium and pubis)
   - Femur: Two
   - Tibia and Fibula: Two (in each leg)
6. *Foot bones (in left and right foot):*
   - Calcaneum: Two
   - Talus: Two
   - Metatarsal: Five + Five (five in each foot)
   - Phalanges: Three phalanges (in each toe except the great toe—proximal, middle and distal, the great toe has two phalanges only—proximal and distal.

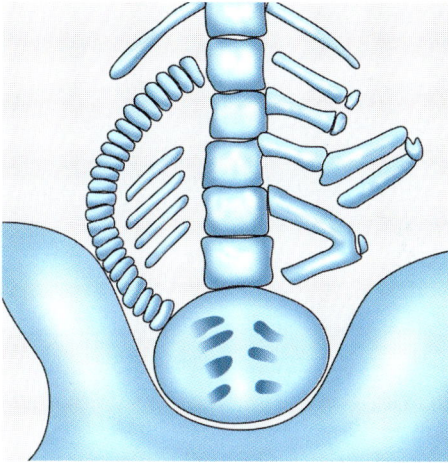

Figure 16.26: Pregnancy

7. *Vertebra column comprises of:*
   Cervical vertebrae: Seven
   Thoracic vertebrae: Twelve
   Lumbar vertebrae: Five
8. *Sternum and ribs:*
   - Sternum has manubrium sterni and four body segments (i.e. sternebra)
   - Ribs: Twenty-four in number (12 ribs on each side of thoracic cage).

PRIMARY OSSIFICATION CENTERS APPEAR IN SKULL IN 7TH OR 8TH PRENATAL WEEK

1. *Cranial bones*
   - Frontal: Two centers
   - Parietal: Two centers
   - Temporal: Several centers (squamous, tympanic, styloid part; petrous part; mastoid part) (ear ossicles; malleus, incus, stapes)

- Ethmoid: Three centers—one for each perpendicular plate and one for each labyrinth
- Sphenoid: Several centers (central: body and lesser wing; right and left, lateral (greater wing and pterygoid process)
- Occipital: Several centers (squamous, condylar, lateral and basilar part)

2. *Facial bones*
   - Nasal
   - Maxilla: One center (in each but additional centers appear in its anterior part).
   - Zygomatic: One ossification center
   - Palatine: One center
   - Lacrimal: One center
   - Inferior nasal conchae: One center
   - Mandible: Membranous and cartilaginous ossification. Each half of the bone is formed from one center in 6 weeks IUL and appearance of the mental foramen
   - Vomer: One center.

3. *Hyoid bone*: Hyoid bone is ossified from six centers. One center appears in each greater carnua towards the end of fetal life.

Hyoid Bone

In elderly age, hyoid bone is a U-shaped bone suspended from the tips of styloid process of two temporal bones by stylohyoid ligaments and lies in the front of the neck between the chin and thyroid cartilage at the level of third cervical vertebra posteriorly. In younger age group, the hyoid bone is in three parts (i.e. one body and two greater cornuae).

Upper Limb Bones (pectoral girdle)

- *Collar bone*: Six weeks IUL (two centers appear in shaft and soon fuse with each other)·
- *Scapula*: Eight weeks IUL (center appears in the body)
- *Humerus*: Eight week (center appears in the shaft)
- *Radius and ulna*: Eight weeks each (forearm bones)

Hand and Finger Bones

- Metacarpals: 9 weeks
- Phalanges:
  - Proximal: 10 weeks
  - Middle: Twelve weeks
  - Distal: Eight weeks

Lower Limb Bones (pelvic girdle)

- Hip bone:
  Ilium: Eight weeks IUL
  Pubis: Two weeks IUL
  Ischium: Sixteen weeks IUL
- Femur: Seven weeks IUL (in shaft)

Leg Bones

- Tibia: Seven weeks IUL
- Fibula: Eight weeks IUL

Foot Bones

- Calcaneum: Third month
- Talus: Sixth month
- Metatarsals: Ninth or tenth month
- Phalanges: Seventh to fifteenth week.

Vertebral Column

Each vertebra has three primary center: one center in the body, one on each half of neural arch (centers appears between 9 and 12 weeks IUL).

Sternum

- Manubrium sterni: 1 to 3 centers
- Sternebra (four): One or two centers in each sternebra (i.e. sternal body segments): Fifth month IUL.

Ribs

24 in number (12 ribs on each side of thoracic cage).

5

Radiographic Positioning, Identification and Radiology in Bone Injuries

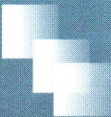

Chapter 17

Radiographic Positioning, Identification and Radiology in Bone Injuries

RADIOGRAPHIC POSITIONING

- *Erect:* Standing or sitting up
- *Supine:* Lying on the back with face upwards
- *Prone:* Lying on the abdomen with face downwards
- *Lateral:* Lying on left or right side that side is placed close to the film (cassette)
- *Oblique:* Turned a little so that the body part is between prone and supine position
- *Right posterior oblique (RPO):* Right posterior side next to the cassette (film)
- *Left posterior oblique (LPO):* Left posterior side near the film (cassette)
- *Right anterior oblique (RAO):* Right anterior side close to the film (cassette)
- *Left anterior oblique (LAO):* Left anterior side close to the film (cassette)
- *Anteroposterior (AP):* X-ray beam enters the posterior surface

- *Posteroanterior (PA)*: X-ray beam enters the posterior surface
- *Lateral:* X-ray beam enters the left side of the body
- *Oblique:* (A) Right AP oblique projection and (B) Left AP oblique projection

In radiological positioning, the proper replacement of persons body part on a cassette to give an accurate image.

IMPORTANT CONSIDERATIONS

To be taken:
1. Anteroposterior/posteroanterior and lateral projection— For depth of foreign bodies, e.g. bullets in a case of forearm injuries.
2. The entire bone should be projected on radiograph.
3. The part should be placed at right angles to the caste.
4. Clothing should be removed from the areas to be radiographed.

POSITIONING OF THE PART

1. *Chest*: Anteroposterior (AP) and lateral
   - Lungs and heart
   - Ribs: Oblique AP
   - Chest: AP infants
2. *Abdomen*: Anteroposterior (AP) and lateral
   - General
   - Urinary tract
   - Gallbladder
   - Pregnancy (in female)—Posteroanterior (PA)
3. *Head*:
   - X-ray of skull: PA and lateral
   - Sinuses and face: PA
   - Mandible: PA and oblique lateral

4. *Vertebral column*:
   - Cervical spine: PA/lateral and oblique.
   - Thoracic spine: AP and lateral
   - Lumbar spine: AP and lateral
   - Sacrum: AP
5. *Arm (pectoral girdle)*:
   - Clavicle: AP
   - Scapula: AP/Lateral
   - Shoulder: AP/Lateral
   - Humerus: AP/Lateral
   - Elbow: AP/Lateral
   - Forearm: AP/Lateral
   - Wrist: PA/Lateral
   - Hand: PA/Oblique
     - Thumb: AP/Lateral
     - Finger: Lateral (single)
6. *Leg (pelvic girdle)*:
   - Pelvis: AP
     - Hip joints: AP/lateral
   - Femur: AP/lateral
   - Knee: AP/lateral
     - Knee intercondylar space
     - Patella
   - Leg: AP/lateral
   - Ankle: AP/internal oblique/external oblique
   - Foot and toes: AP/lateral/ AP oblique/ PA oblique
   - Heel
   - Pelvis and hip joints (in infants and small children): AP.

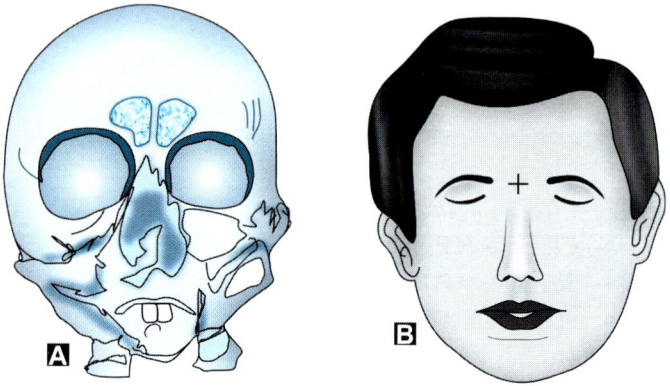

Figures 17.1A and B: Skull: Anteroposterior (AP)–Supine

SKULL: ANTEROPOSTERIOR (AP)–SUPINE (FIGS 17.1A AND B)

- Patient's head should be raised on a foam rubber pad.
- Remove denture, hairpins, etc. from scalp hair.
- Center to the nasion (root of the nose) between the eyes.

CHEST (FIGS 17.2A AND B)

- Patient's shoulders are pressed forward.
- Patient to be told to breathe in deeply and hold the breathe.
- Tell the patient to breathe in deeply and hold the breathe.
- Lower part of diaphragm should be visible.

KNEE (FIGS 17.3A AND B)

- Knee joint fully extended and foot is placed in inverted position.

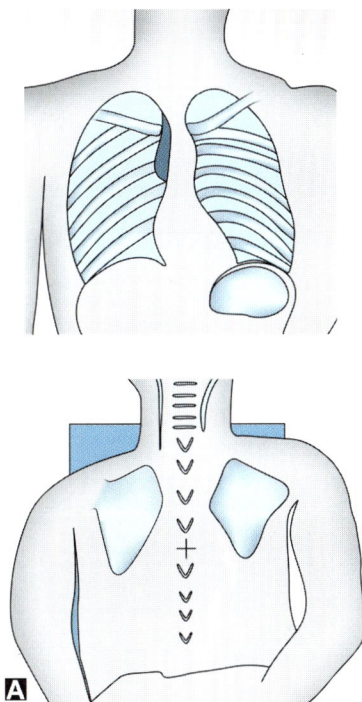

Figure 17.2A: Chest PA—Standing erect

- Cassette is placed lengthwise under the knee.
- Knee joint is fully extended and elevated.
- Cassette is placed lengthwise below the knee.
- Turning on the right or left side.

IDENTIFICATION FROM RADIOLOGICAL EXAMINATIONS

Radiological studies are helpful from comparison studies to establish identity.

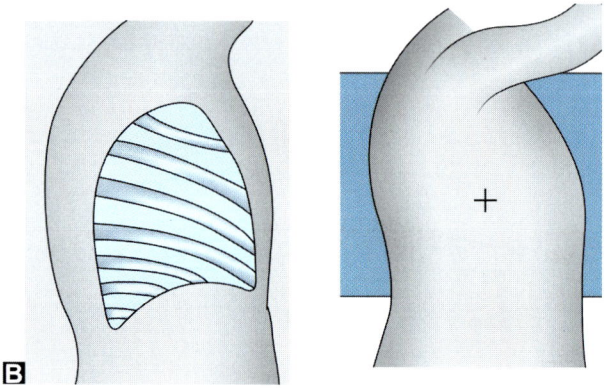

Figure 17.2B: Chest lateral left—standing erect

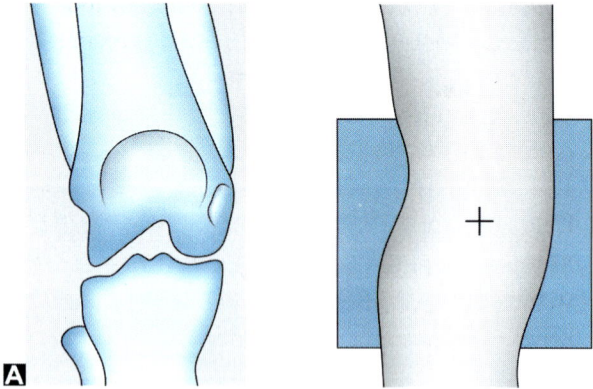

Figure 17.3A: Anteroposterior projection of the knee (Supine)

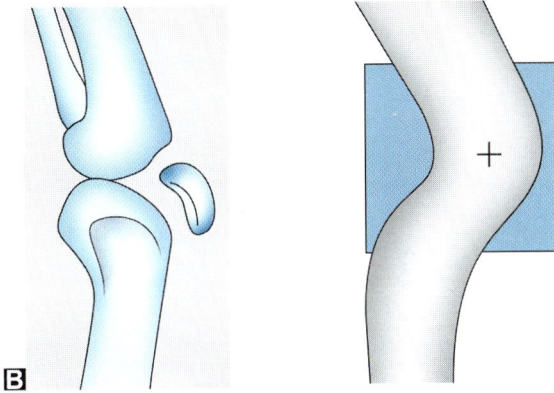

Figure 17.3B: Lateral projection of the knee

- Antemortem and postmortem radiographs when available for companion of similarities and differences.
- Over-riding canine tooth or central incisor tooth; supernumerary tooth, i.e. extratooth, when present is helpful in identity.
- Bone trabecular and nutritional canals show individual pattern of the person to establish identification (Figs 17.4A to C).
- Degenerative hypertrophic changes in the margins of vertebrae in the form of lipping, spurring and osteophyte formations revealed on radiological examinations are helpful in identification.
- Nasal cavity, maxillary antrum and sella turica also show individual variability which are helpful in establishing personal identity.

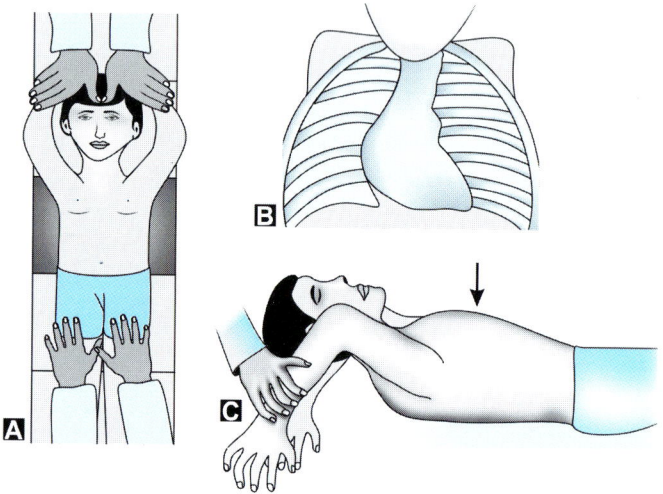

Figures 17.4A to C: Infant supporting parents must wear lead apron and lead gloves

- Comparison of frontal sinuses — antemortem or post-mortem skull fragments of frontal area reveal distinctive pattern of airspaces, their margins, septa and labulated pattern and other close surroundings help in establishing personal identity (even in identical twins frontal sinuses patterns are different). The paranasal sinuses — frontal sinuses and maxillary antra expand and develop during adolescence and reach to the maximum size during adult age (In 5% population the frontal sinuses are absent and are not developed).
- Harris' lines (growth lines) in the distal end of the shaft of humerus are helpful in identity as no two individuals have the same ridge pattern (Fig. 17.5).

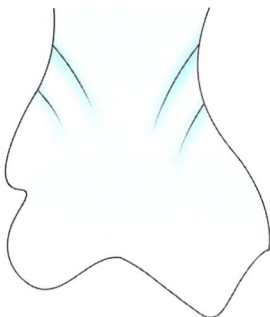

Figure 17.5: Harris' lines (growth lines) in the distal end of the shaft of humerus

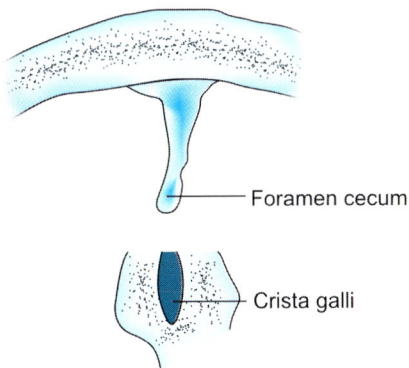

Foramen cecum

Crista galli

Figure 17.6: Cribriform plate of ethmoid bone

• Trabecular pattern, vascular grooves and other helpful findings like crista galli, cribriform plate of ethmoid bone and foramen cecum help in identification of the fragment and comparison helps in identification (Fig. 17.6).

- In bundle of bones or bone fragments when recovered a healed fracture in the shaft of a collar bone or forearm bone (radius) showing residual defect from healing of fractured bone with intact plates and screws also establish positive identification of a person from studying the earlier records of hospital treatment and X-ray examinations.
- In mass casualty, i.e. aircraft accidents—burnt, charred and fragmented bodies, railroad accidents showing mutilated parts of the body; natural disorders— earthquakes, floods collapse of building; fire accidents and in bomb explosions a large number of persons are involved requiring identification.
- Dental radiological studies done earlier prior to death when comparison of antemortem and postmortem dental studies done to establish personal identity.

Disarticulated lower jaw and resected upper jaw from the dead during postmortem examination are used to establish the identity of the person. Dental records are also helpful in many a times. Burnt teeth are also useful in giving information about the burning. Gray side of burnt tooth indicates the labial side and exposure to intense heat and burning (i.e. complete combustion) and whereas black side of tooth is indicative of lingual side. Age of the person can be estimated from dental eruption of temporary and permanent teeth. Eruption of 1st permanent molar in children and third molar in adult lower jaw is also helpful in age determination. Radiological studies are helpful in these cases. Dental radiology is helpful in aggressive teeth bite crimes as women and children in sexual assaults, criminal violence and child abuse, teeth are used as weapons in criminal assaults and physical altercations. Bitemarks of frontal teeth on skin of female breast, body and buttocks are found in the form of two curved broken lines opposing each other in elliptical form. Swaps are taken for studies of saliva to establish the identity of the accused. The photographs are also taken to preserve the evidence which corrilate with X-ray dental images.

- Bones burnt intensely with intact flesh in incineration and house-burning show shrinkage and cracks perpendicular to the long axis of the burnt bone. Dry bones without flesh on intense burning show longitudinal cracks.
- When temperature and heat is intense like in incineration or funeral fire, the bones are grayish-white in color and more fragile but retain their configuration. They can be used for comparison identification.
- The positioning of the fragmentary remains, are important for the study of these patterns radiographically.
- The lower four incisor teeth show pulp chamber (PC) and root canal (RC). Incisors, canines, lower premolars have a single tapering root with single root canal (Figs 17.7A and B). They can be visualized by taking dental X-rays. The pulp chambers and root canals became narrow with age (Fig 17.8).
- Deciduous teeth are 20 in number and permanent teeth 32.

RADIOLOGY IN BONY INJURIES

Bony injuries to the body skeleton are best studied on Radiological examinations. In the dead, postmortem

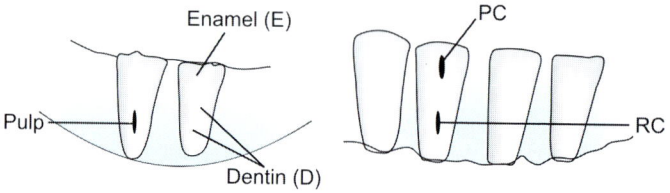

Figures 17.7A and B: (A) Lower Incisor showing pulp cavity (PC), (B) Root canal (RC) helpful in age and Identity

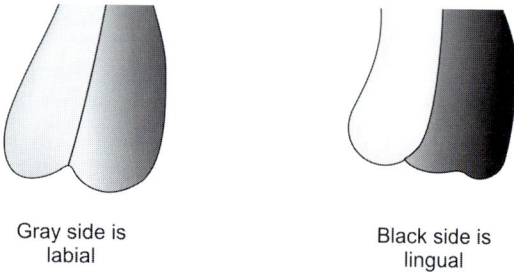

Gray side is labial

Black side is lingual

Figure 17.8: Burnt teeth (house burning)

examination reveals various aspects of fractures. Their location, type of fracture, direction of force acting locally, accidental or inflicted. The point of impact; weapon or an object causing it also can be made out. In traffic accidents a pedestrian sustains a typical injury known as 'bumper fracture' at the knee joints; little above on thighs (femur) or below on legs (tibia and fibula) bilateral and symmetrical. X-ray examination of AP/PA and lateral views are taken to know the nature of fracture.

Wedge-shaped fracture of tibia (bumper injury) in a pedestrian met with the traffic accident (Fig. 17.9). The X-ray shows forward displacement of the bone fragment. The base of the triangular fragment of bone indicates the

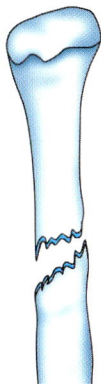

Figure 17.9: Wedge-shaped fracture of tibia

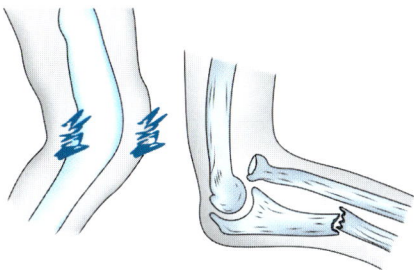

Figure 17.10: Fracture of ulna

site of impact and the apex of the fragment points in the direction in which the vehicle was traveling. In children, bumper fracture is in the femur. Forearm injuries are sustained in defending himself to save from the attack and ward off the blow by raising the forearm. In this attack, the ulna is broken resulting in bending fracture of ulna (Fig. 17.10).

In violent asphyxial deaths, the superior horns of thyroid cartilage and greater cornuae of hyoid bone are fractured in throttling greater cornua of hyoid bone are fractured at the junction of inner two-thirds and outer one-third. In thyroid cartilage, commonly one or both superior horns are fractured in strangulation (Figs 17.11 and 17.12).

CHILD ABUSE

Child abuse is mostly under three years of age. Bony injuries are common due to repeated beating. Antero-posterior and lateral views of X-rays reveal various

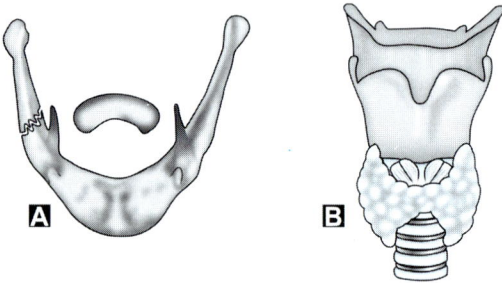

Figures 17.11A and B: (A) Fracture of hyoid bone from manual/ strangulation (throttling); (B) Fracture of superior cornua of thyroid cartilage from strangulation

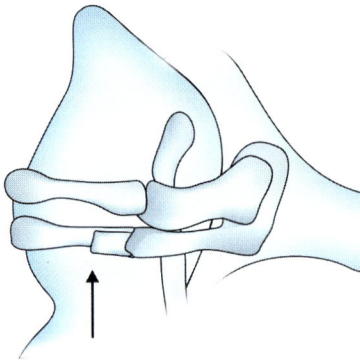

Figure 17.12: Fracture of greater cornuae of hyoid bone

fractures of skeleton and dislocations of joints. Often the upper or lower limbs are grabed and the child is shaken or pulled and also swung. The fractures of long bones of limbs are most common. Collar bones are also fractured in their middle-third in their shaft. The ribs of thoracic cage are fractured from direct trauma. Diaphyses of long bones show transverse, oblique; spiral fractures which are seen in X-ray examinations. Bilateral metaphyseal fractures and proximal phalanx of hands are also fractured. Periosteum of long bones gets separated from pulling and twisting injuries causing subperiosteal hematoma with calcification around the shaft of limb bones are seen in radiological studies of child abuse. Epiphyseal separations are common in traction injuries. Before antopsy the entire body of the dead child should be subjected to radiological examinations as they reveal physical abuse of the child shoulder girdle injuries are sustained due to grabbing with upper limbs and the child is swung. Bilateral injuries are common at growing ends of long bones. Scapula also may be fractured in its body being the flat thin bone—metaphyseal injuries with fractures are common in knee joints, ankle joints and in lower end of humerus. Dislocation of joints occurs from local forceful injuries (Figs 17.13 to 17.20). Rib fractures are common in child abuse. Anteroposterior compression causes fractures in midaxillary line and paravertebral line (i.e. posterior fractures of ribs) and anterior fractures in costochondral junctions, on radiological examination. The posterior fractures in paravertebral line show different ages of healing indicating that the injuries were inflicted at different periods. Skull fractures are also inflicted by blunt force and forcible impacts against the head from dashing against a wall or wooden furniture. Severe injuries cause intracranial hemorrhages. Fissure fractures of skull are common. Pond fractures of skull may also occur. Subdural and subarachnoid hemorrhages occur from shearing forces which act on the brain.

- CT is preferable for subarachnoid hemorrhage.
- MRI is better to detect subdural hemorrhage.
- CT and MRI are used to detect epidural hemorrhage.

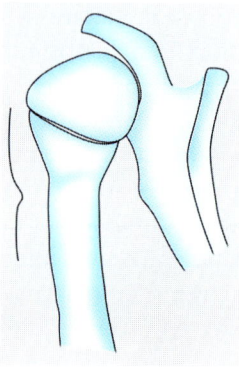

Figure 17.13: Fracture neck of humerus

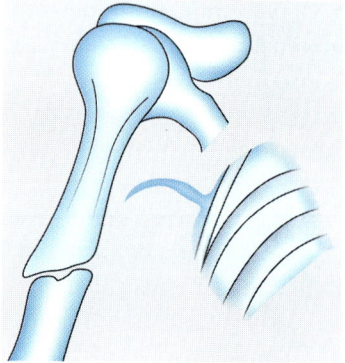

Figure 17.14: Fracture middle shaft of humerus

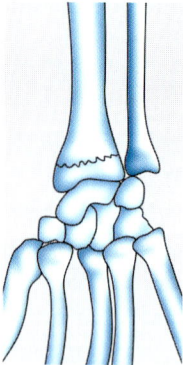

Figure 17.15: Colles' fracture (wrist)

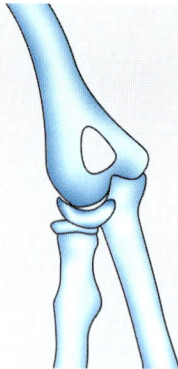

Figure 17.16: Fracture dislocation of elbow joint

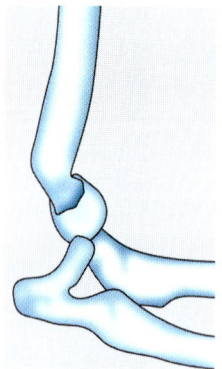

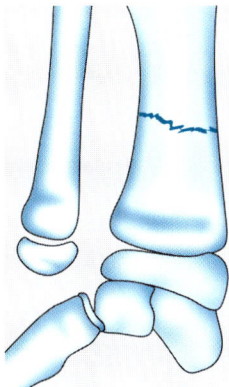

Figure 17.17: Green stick fracture of radius (Forearm)

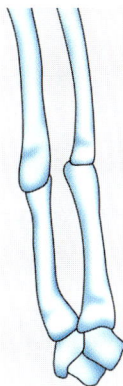

Figure 17.18: Fracture of shafts of ulna and radius in forearm

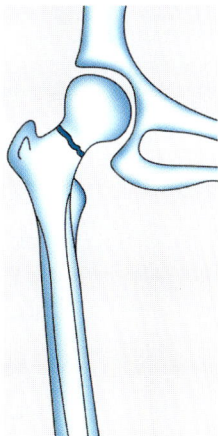

Figure 17.19: Fracture— neck of femur

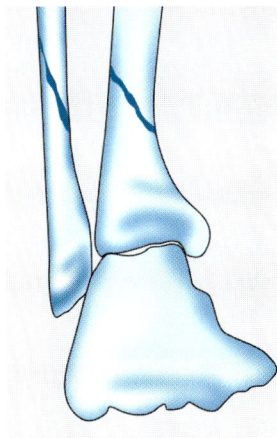

Figure 17.20: Anteroposterior view—fractures of tibia and fibula

- CT is also used to defect fractures of skull.
- CT discloses fractures of ribs which are not visible in X-ray examinations.
- CT is of value in injuries to the thoracic and abdominal viscera.
- Ultrasound is of value in injuries to abdominal viscera and retroperitoneal organs when injured.
- Girl child is sexually abused.
- Shaking injuries cause subdural hemorrhage when shaken by holding shoulders, arms and scalp hair. In these cases, rotational force causes tearing of bridging veins.
- Fist blows and kicks over lower thoracic and upper abdomen produce rupture of liver, tearing of mesentery and perforation of small intestine.
- Gripmarks are found around elbows and ankles when the child is held and hurled into a cot.
- Teeth bitemarks on face, chest and limbs are found from biting.
- Cigarette burns are common on soles of feet.

BATTERING OF WIFE (SPOUSAL ABUSE)

Battering of wife is a common domestic violence all over the world. The injuries sustained are not accidental. Fist blows are common. Abrasions, contusions and lacerated wounds are common. Swelling on face against lower jaw due to contusion is common.

Injuries against the chin and teeth cause fracture—dislocations of teeth. Fracture of lower jaw may occur at the body and angle of jaw. Nasal bones are also fractured.

Radiological examinations reveal fractures. Skin and soft tissue injuries in the form of finger imprints in the form of patterned contusion are seen on side of face.

ABUSE ON OLD AND ELDERLY PERSONS

They suffer from ill treatment by inflicting fist blows and kicks, pushing against the ground. Lower jaw is fractured from blunt force injury at the level of mental foramen and at deep socket of canine tooth. X-ray reveal fractures and are economical. CT and MRI are more useful but costly.

6

Radiology and Firearm Injuries

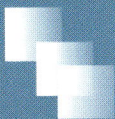

Chapter 18

Firearm Injuries

Radiological examination is very important in every case of death by firing using a gun to commit the crime. It is always better to subject the dead body for X-ray examination before the postmortem examination. A bullet or several bullets may be revealed in side deep into the body cavities in internal organs and skeleton parts of the body. X-ray examination becomes more important when only the wounds of entrance are present externally or skin surface and the exit wounds are absent. In most of the firing deaths the missile (bullet or pellet) is found underneath the skin in intercostal space and closer to the vertebral column. The X-ray examination reveals the number, direction, bone splintering and also the nature of the firearm. Bullet of rifled firearm looses its velocity of spin and rotation on striking a bone or resistance from the tissues inside the body. Exit wound is not produced due to loss of velocity and the bullet comes to rest even in muscles. Anteroposterior and lateral views are essential, missiles (bullets and pellets) are seen as opaque foreign body images on the X-ray film deep inside the body. In the absence of exit wounds, it becomes essentials to subject the entire body to X-ray examination and then only the body is disposed after postmortem examination. In decomposed skeletonizing body and in case of exhumed body X-ray examination with a view to detect bullets or pellets when the history of firing with a gun is available. Examination of clothing worn by the deceased when available on exhumation also reveals gun powder residue and small perforations around the large perforation on holding against sunlight and then examination.

These minute perforations on clothing are due to burnt and partly burnt grains of gun powder. Recovery of bullets or pellets confirm the use of firearm (gun) and death from firearm injury. It has been seen a dead body revealed a large lead ball indicating the use of a muzzleloader smooth bore country made gun or a 0.410 musket used by police and railway protection force. Along with the missile when the firearm is also recovered the crime investigation becomes easier. Test bullet and crime bullet are examined using a comparison microscope. Fragmentation of lead bullets (non jacketed) may occur and seen as taking the X-ray. Lead is soft metalloid and lead bullets are opaque on radiological examination. As the base metal of a bullet is lead which is soft and make it hard antimony or tin is added to make them hardened lead bullets. These bullets may be covered partly or fully by a copper or cupronickel (copper alloy). These bullets are known as jacketed bullets. These bullets also cause opaque shadows on the X-ray films when taken in shooting death. In partially covered bullets the tip is exposed. On firing, the metal jacket may get separated inside the body. The separated jacket can be identified on taking the X-ray. It is often confused for a second bullet.

The metal casing has lower radiodensity than the lead and hardened lead alloy. In such cases, rifling marks are seen or metal jacket which is separated and not on the lead bullet inside. The separated jacket casing is recovered and preserved during postmortem examination. For examination of rifling marks, mushrooming and flattening of the exposed tip on hitting a bone inside the body brokes the bone into multiple fragments. The multiple bone fragments from braking of the bone is also visualized an X-ray examination.

The broken bone fragments individually act as projectiles and cause greater tissue damage. Extensive fracturing of skull occurs in bullet or pellet injuries from the firearm in contact or close range to the head. The revolving rifle bullet (service rifle bullet with 3000 revolutions per second) may drill into the skull and produce a small rounded punched out hole in the outer table of skull and on the opposite side a large, irregular beveled hole on X-ray of the head (skull). The bullet is not found inside the skull cavity as it has escaped from the exit hole making tract inside the brain and its meninges (Figs 18.1 and 18.2). Pellet injuries as smooth bore gun causes bursting type of fractures of skull with scattering of brain tissue outside the skull cavity is produced. Detached isolated ear in the injury may be found sticking on the opposite side of the wall little away from the injured at the scene.

Bursting type of fracture is produced from the compact mass of pellets at contact or close range. The near and distant ranges dispersion of pellets produce individual pellet holes on skin and soft tissues on the person.

The 'Birdshot' cartridge of smooth bore gun (12 bore gun) contains small dust pellets and the "Buckshot" cartridge contains nine large pellets. Radiological

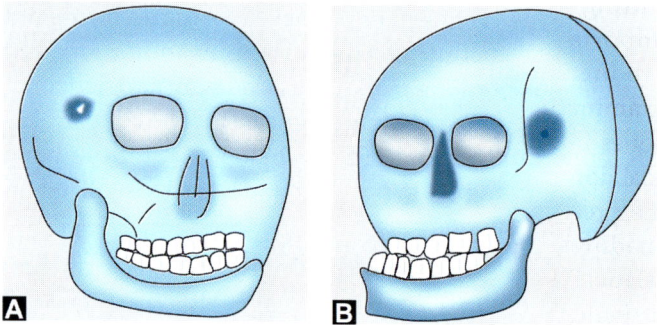

Figures 18.1A and B: Bullet injury to head from rifled firearm. (A) Entry hole in the skull (right temple) is small, rounded with clean cut margins; (B) Exit hole in skull (left temple) is large beveled and irregular

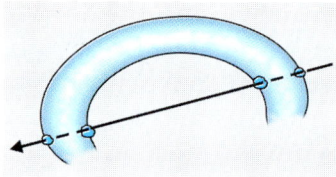

Figure 18.2: Punch out and beveled hole in the skull

examination of these victius confirm the use of certain type of cartridge used in firing from a 12-bore gun very close or from a distance range. Suicidal firearm injuries can be made out as they are confined to locations and sites of selection (election) and on easily accessible parts of the body and head. On the head and face, the right temple and center of forehead are the common sites (Figs 18.4 and 18.5).

Other sites are left side of chest as procardia, epigastrium (pit of stomach) and the pit of neck (suprasternal).

During autopsy recovery of bullets or pellets is very important as it helps in detection of crime and in production of evidence similar to X-ray images. CT examination is also helpful in fragmentation of skull bones in bullet and pellet injuries. The chest and thoracoabdominal injuries on radiological examination reveal the presence of missiles (bullets and pellets) as opaque shadows under the dooms of diaphragm and also in relation to the spinal column. In an X-ray film widespread of pellets from dispersal indicates the firining from a distance. The `billiard ball' effect also may be seen from striking these pellets with one another and spreading in the wide area giving a false impression of long range firing. Examination of clothing worn by the decreased at the time of firing is also as important as the dead body itself from firearm injury.

a. Birdshot injury produced by dust pellets = X-ray of chest showing shot pattern of dust pellets in wide area from their spread (Figs 18.3A and 18.7A to C).

b. Buckshot injury: X-ray shows widespread of 9 large shots dispersing inside (Fig 18.3B and 18.8A to C).

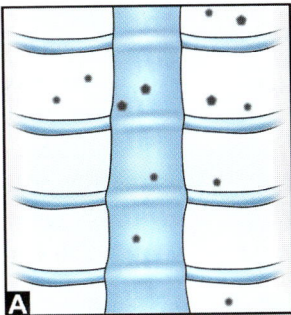

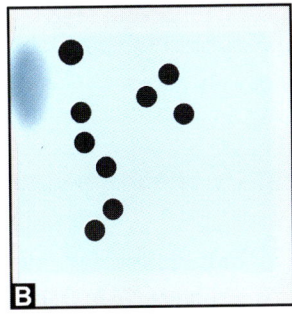

Figures 18.3A and B: (A) Birdshot injury; (B) Buckshot injury

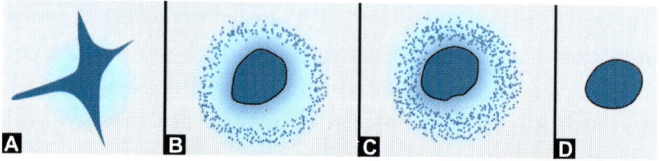

Figures 18.4A to D: Injuries sustained from rifle at different ranges; (A) Contact shot; (B) Close shot (1 to 6 inches); (C) Near shot; (D) Distant shot (12 inches and above)

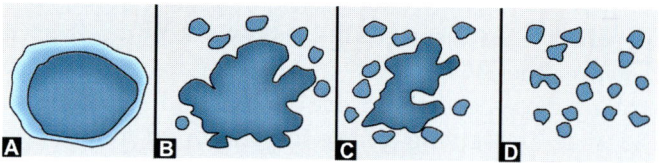

Figures 18.5A to D: Injuries sustained from shotgun at different ranges (A) At a range of up to 1 yard; (B) At a range of up to 1-2 yards; (C) At a range of up to 2-4 yards; (D) At a range above 4 yards

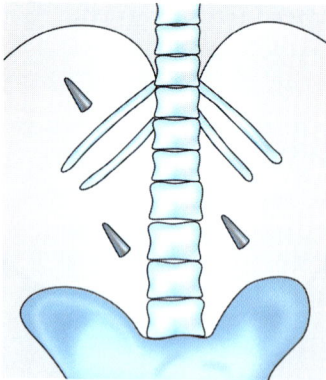

Figure 18.6: Rifled firearm injuries showing bullets and their direction

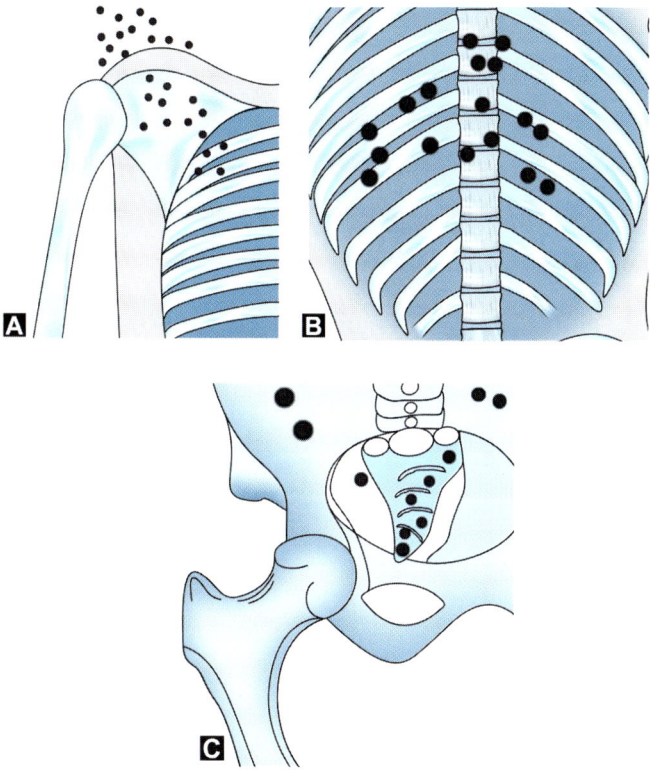

Figures 18.7A to C: (A) 'Birdshot' injury (dust size nearly 2600 small pellets) in the cartridge; (B and C) 'Buckshot' injury (9 large pellets in the cartridge). (Each pellet is 6 to 8 mm in diameter)

Radiographs (X-rays) of the dead from shooting with a firearm show pellets or bullets in MLC form the best evidence in the investigation and in the trial of the case in court of law (Fig 18.6).

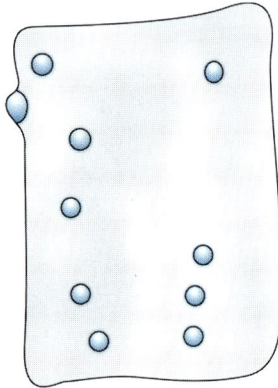

Figures 18.8A: Buck shot injury from 9 yards distance: Satelite pellet produced WE above the right nipple

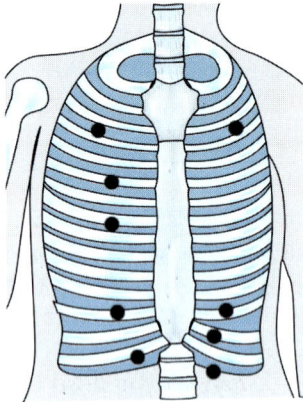

Figure 18.8B

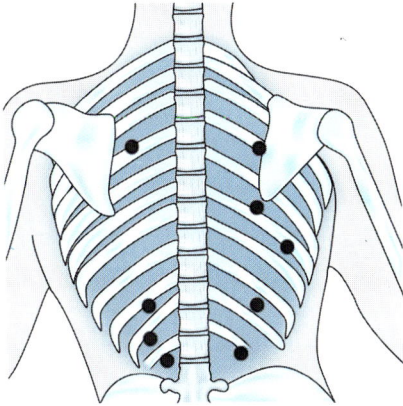

Figure 18.8C

Figures 18.8B and C: Buckshot injury

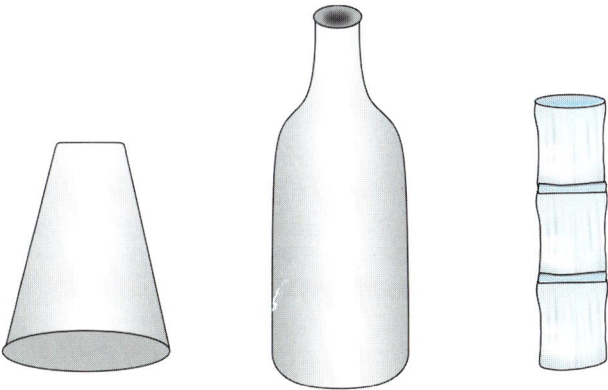

Figure 18.9: A glass tumbler, a beer bottle, or a piece of bamboo-stick may be forcibly introduced into the victim of Sodomy. They can be detected on X-ray examinations

FOREIGN BODIES SEEN IN X-RAY

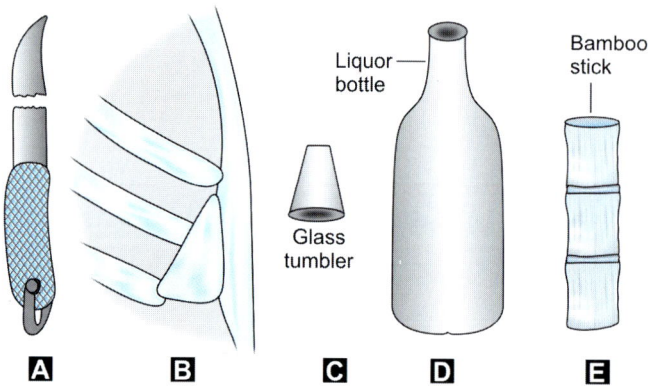

Figures 18.10A to D: (A) Snapped knife (Tip is retained in the skull cavity); (B) Broken glass piece in chest wall; (C) Glass tumbler inside vagina of female; (D) Liquor bottle introduced into rectum forcibly; (E) Bamboo-stick is also introduced but rare

OTHER FOREIGN BODIES VISUALIZED IN RADIOGRAPHS (FIGS 18.9 AND 18.10)

- Most of the foreign bodies are radiopaque on X-ray studies.
- The broken tip of a knife, on forcible stabbing on the head and skull.
- A broken piece of transparent glass in the chest wall on stabbing or a broken piece from a broken beer bottle used for stabbing in criminal assaults.
- Metal fragments, i.e. sharpnels in bomb explosion casting opaque shadows on X-rays examination.
- Foreign body insertions on forcible thrusts into the vagina and rectum are common in psychiatric cases of sexual abuse.

Index